THE 10 DAY SUGAR DETOX CHALLENGE

The Ultimate Guide to Reset the Brain, Eliminate Sugar Cravings, and Break Sugar Addiction to Burn Fat and Lose Weight
(30 Anti-Inflammatory Recipes Included)

Silvana Siskov

Thank you for purchasing "The 10 Day Sugar Detox Challenge"

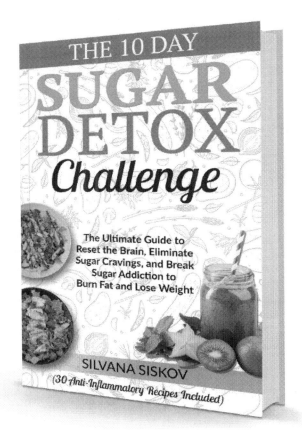

To get the most out of the book, download the free Workbook at bit.ly/sugar-detox-workbook

THE 10 DAY SUGAR DETOX CHALLENGE

Table of Contents

Introduction

There is a serious crisis currently happening that doesn't get reported on the news, but it's threatening the health of the developed world. It's the sugar crisis.

Something that we have been enjoying for generations has become detrimental to our health, and turning into a public health crisis. There are many reasons for this. Sugar consumption has increased dramatically over the last 50 years, and its damaging effects are highly noticeable. The health care system is overwhelmed by the treatment of the damage that sugar causes to our bodies. As you may already be aware, a large sugar intake often leads to obesity, various other health conditions, and even death.

Sugar is a naturally occurring carbohydrate found in many plant-based foods. The body converts it into glucose, and its role in nutrition is to provide fuel and short-term energy.

If your sugar intake was derived from natural sources such as fruit or vegetables, your body wouldn't have a problem with it. In fact, it would benefit from it because these ingredients include vitamins, fibre, minerals, and phytochemicals. They all play a positive role in nutrition, supporting your body to break the glucose down gradually.

It is important to remember that sugar is dangerous when refined as all the extra nutrients are stripped away. In which case, you're taking in pure sugar that acts similar to a drug.

Refined sugar, found in many processed foods, creates an imbalance of the blood sugar levels and causes chaos with the hormones and neurotransmitters, plunging you into a cycle of highs and lows. This results in cravings for more sugar to bring you back to the next high. At the same time, the excess glucose in your system causes insulin overproduction, which stores fat in your cells. This process can lead to many health issues ranging from obesity and type 2 diabetes to developing memory problems.

When people think of refined sugar, they mainly associate it with table sugar added to teas or coffees. Some people don't find it too difficult to cut out, and perhaps you've already done that. The trouble is that sugar is an ingredient used in many processed and packaged foods. The food industry uses a very wide collection of names for it — over 80. Later in the book, I will give more details about identifying sugar and how to find it when it isn't clearly labelled on packaging.

To break the cycle of sugar addiction and the associated health hazards, you'll need to learn how to leave it out of your diet without damaging your nutrition or pleasure when eating.

Let's look at a few vital facts to help you understand the danger of sugar and the ways it affects us:

- Sugar is found in many processed foods, even those that aren't sweet.
- A US study in 2016[1] showed that children in the US

eat around three times the recommended daily allowance — while another US study in 2018[2] found that toddlers under two were consuming almost the recommended amount for an adult woman.

- Charity Diabetes UK reports[3] that more than 4.9 million people in the UK suffer from sugar-related diseases, with another 13.6 million at increased risk of type 2 diabetes.
- In the USA, the National Diabetes Statistics Report,[4] 2000, found that 34.2 million (over 10%) have diabetes, while 88 million (over 30%) are prediabetic.
- In 2002, it was reported that most adults in the UK were overweight, and one in five was obese. Thirty thousand deaths a year were attributed to obesity.[5] As sugar is a leading cause of obesity, it indicates that sugar is a significant contributor to death.
- The obesity level was 42.4% in the USA in 2018, with severe obesity at 9.2%.[6]
- Refined sugar is more addictive than cocaine.[7]

Numerous studies have been carried out, all showing the danger of high sugar consumption to your health.

The aim of this book is to provide you with the important information you need to make healthy lifestyle choices, and to explain, teach, and show you how you can live a sugar-free life.

If you want to start eating healthily but don't know how, and if you've been trying to stop eating sugar but cannot quit, this book is for you.

I am proud to be able to share my knowledge and expertise with you while you go through this process and guide you through your challenges over the next ten days. In this practical 10 Day programme, you will receive all the guidance you need to get your sugar cravings under control and enjoy better health.

Each chapter of this book represents one day of your 10 Day challenge. Chapter One will be your first day; Chapter Two will be your second day, etc.

At the end of each day, you will be given a task to complete. I suggest you complete the tasks to get the maximum health benefits from this book.

The knowledge you gain will improve many areas of your life. You will learn the importance of mindful eating, receive valuable advice and information that can easily be applied in your everyday life, get recipes for sugar-free meals, break your addiction, and much more. Throughout the book, you will be encouraged to take actionable steps which will help you improve your bad eating habits, burn fat, and lose excess weight.

I strongly recommend downloading *The 10 Day Sugar Detox Challenge Workbook* by going to bit.ly/sugar-detox-workbook. The Workbook accompanies this book and offers additional support on your journey. You will find all the tasks you need to do at the end of each day, from Day One to Day Ten. Your commitment to completing these tasks will play an essential role in your success.

I'm not saying that going sugar-free will be a simple task, but this book and the Workbook are designed to provide you with enough guidance and information about quitting sugar the easy way in only ten days.

All you need to do is commit to the process and follow the guidance in this book. If you follow my advice, your sugar-free journey won't end with the last page of this book.

In only a few short days, you'll be able to identify where sugar can be found and how to create a healthy diet plan that can lead to more energy, better physical health, and increased mental clarity. No more feeling lethargic, ruining your health because of bad habits, or experiencing brain fog.

The book is packed with valuable information, giving you the knowledge that will make a real difference on the road to living without sugar and set you up to continue your journey.

As a nutritionist and health coach, I have supported many clients over the years and helped them change their unhealthy eating habits. They have developed new and healthy behaviours that led them to overcome sugar cravings, achieve better health, and experience improved well-being.

As I discussed earlier, the sugar crisis needs to be tackled worldwide, but the only person you can help directly is yourself. Therefore, the next ten days will be crucial. It will challenge you mentally and emotionally. You may experience some adverse side effects due to sugar withdrawal from your diet. But trust me, it will all be worth it in the end.

Ten days is a short period of time considering that this programme will change your life, so I'm encouraging you to show your full commitment and enjoy the health benefits for the rest of your life.

Your health is in your hands, and the time to start the sugar detox challenge is now.

Are you ready for your transformation?

Are you ready to break the sugar addiction and take control of your health?

Let the journey begin.

Chapter 1

Day One: Getting to Know About Sugar and Its Dangers

Welcome to Day One of the Sugar Detox Challenge!

Why am I writing this book?

About 20 years ago, I was addicted to sugar. This addiction lasted for several years. I needed to have sugary foods every single day, several times a day. Chocolate bars were my biggest weakness. I needed them. I wanted them. I couldn't live without them. I was not in control of my food. Food was controlling me.

My love for chocolates, or obsession, kept me in a vicious cycle of bingeing on chocolate several times a day and doing vigorous exercises following each binging episode to burn them off. I didn't understand at the time that my eating habits were very unhealthy.

Years later, when I started to show interest in good nutrition due to my tiredness, irritability, and so on, I knew it was the time to break my addictive patterns and change my eating and lifestyle habits.

This decision made a significant difference, not only in how my body felt but in the way I felt about my body.

In this book, you will learn about the importance of cutting down on sugar.

On the first day of your sugar detox, you will learn about what sugar is and why it is so bad for your health. You'll also be encouraged to search for your *why*. I also suggest you stop eating sugary products today. You may not know about all the foods that contain sugar, as you will learn about them later in the book, but if you follow your intuition and remove the foods from your diet that you believe contain sugar, it is a step in the right direction.

You probably won't feel any effects of your detox at the end of today, apart from possible cravings later in the day. And if you feel hungry, I'd like you to make a healthy choice rather than reaching for unhealthy snacks, or foods loaded with unhealthy fats and simple carbs.

Remember, eating unhealthy won't help you get closer to your goal; it will move you further away from it.

Any long-term habit is hard to change, and changing your diet is no different. Identifying your reasons for quitting or reducing sugar consumption will give you motivation, purpose, and the desire to start cutting sugar out of your diet to reach your goal. And this will be your task to complete at the end of today.

What is Sugar?

So, what is sugar?

I assumed I knew the answer before doing my course in nutrition, but I quickly realised that it was far more complicated than I initially thought.

Perhaps, the question should be, "What are sugars?" because sugar isn't just one thing. It is a type of small carbohydrate molecule. Starch and fibre are also carbohydrates, but they are more complex types. Your digestive system can break down sugar, starch, and fibre to form glucose — the kind of sugar the body uses.

Humans have always eaten sugar in various forms without damaging their health. But over the last few decades, sugar has been proven to be one of the contributing factors for many chronic diseases.

There are various types of sugar with a range of names, which we will explore later in the book.

The simplest types of sugar are monosaccharides and disaccharides. Monosaccharides are glucose, fructose and galactose. They are made up of single sugar molecules and form an essential part of nutrition. They bring many health benefits and are found in fruit and vegetables. When two different types of monosaccharides combine, they form a disaccharide. Examples of disaccharides include sucrose, lactose, and maltose. They are derived from milk, grains, and some fruit and vegetables, and provide the body with a quick energy source.

Sucrose is the sugar you use for your tea, sprinkle on your breakfast cereal or use in baking, and it is derived from two natural sources — sugar cane and sugar beet. The refining process involves stripping the sugar away from all the other elements.

Remember, sugar can be found in a wide variety of fruit and vegetables, dairy products and grains, but as long as it's eaten or drunk along with the natural source, the human body can process it without causing any damage to health.

As you start to learn about sugar, I'd like you to take the first step today and begin eliminating sugar from your diet. At this early stage of the process, whatever your interpretation of sugar and sugary foods is, it is a good starting point to begin creating a change. Any small change you do today can make a big difference in the future. Think of today as a new beginning, and remember that the power is in your hands.

Each day over the next ten days, you'll learn more about sugar and the necessary habits you need to develop to remove sugar from your diet. This will help you to improve your relationship with food and overcome sugar cravings and addiction.

To better understand where sugar came from and how it made its way into the shops and the foods we eat, we need to look through history and go back thousands of years ago.

Sugar cane is believed to have been first cultivated in Polynesia. From here, it spread to India and Iran. After the Persian Empire fell to the Arabic invasion in 642 AD, sugar spread throughout the Islamic empire, reaching as far as Spain. At the end of the 11th century, the Crusaders brought sugar to Europe, but only as a costly luxury.[8] This changed when the refining process for sugar was introduced to Europe, through Venice, in the 15th century. In the same century, the cane was taken to America, where sugar plantations were set up, making sugar more common throughout Europe and America. As you may know, the supply that met the sugar craze was fuelled almost entirely by the slave trade.

It was not until sugar beet was developed in the 18th century that sugar became as common as it is now. The beet, primarily bred from the cane, could grow in European conditions, so prices tumbled. Sugar was available to everyone, and throughout the 19th and 20th centuries, it found its way into every type of food you could imagine.

Why is Sugar Bad for Your Health?

Humans have been consuming sugars from various food items for thousands of years. So, why are health experts now saying that sugar is bad for us?

Let's explore this.

What has changed is the type of sugars and the amount consumed. This will be explored in more detail in later chapters. There's a big difference between natural sugars and free sugars. For example, when you eat an apple, the sugar combined with other nutrients, notably fibre, ensure that the sugar is processed inside the body to protect your health as opposed to damaging it.

However, when the sugar is stripped away and processed (or refined), it no longer contains nutrients that keep your body balanced. The body absorbs all the sugar, and it overwhelms your system. This leads to a high sugar spike in the bloodstream, and when this happens, the pancreas produces insulin to remove the excess sugar from the blood. Insulin is a fat-storage hormone, and regular overeating and unhealthy eating can cause insulin resistance leading to obesity and many illnesses and severe health conditions.

When I first decided to cut refined sugar out of my diet, I didn't think I'd need to give up too many foods, but the more I learned about the nutritional values of various food ingredients, including sugar, I saw my list of forbidden foods increasing.

Not only did I discover the high amount of sugar in cakes and chocolates, but I also noticed that it was hiding in most packaged foods on supermarket shelves. For instance, I used to think that there were plenty of healthy cereals on the market, but I soon discovered that even the most "healthy" cereals were sources of sugar.

High consumption of refined sugars has a wide range of dangerous implications for our health. The most crucial include:

- *Poor dental health*: It is well-known that sugary foods and drinks can cause tooth decay (dental caries).[9] Most attention has traditionally been paid to the effects of sweets and fizzy drinks on children's teeth, but this has also become a significant problem for adult dental health due to the high sugar consumption in the modern diet.[10]
- *Obesity*: While sugar isn't the only culprit in today's

obesity epidemic, it is undoubtedly a major one. As mentioned before, obesity is currently running at 42.4% in the US, with severe obesity at 9.2% [6], and the UK and other developed countries are not far behind. Obesity plays a significant factor in severe health issues, most notably heart disease and stroke.

- *Diabetes*: Cases of type 2 diabetes are also reaching epidemic levels, with over 10% of the US population affected, while over 30% are at serious risk of diabetes. The direct connection between sugar intake and type 2 diabetes is complex, but there's no doubt that obesity, which sugar certainly contributes to, is one of the leading causes of type 2 diabetes.
- *High blood pressure*: Although it's long been known that being overweight or obese could involve a risk of high blood pressure, health professionals have only in recent years proved the impact of high sugar intake on blood pressure.[11] This, in turn, involves a higher risk of cardiovascular disease such as a heart attack.

The above factors are highly damaging to your overall health and well-being. Also, the evidence suggests that sugar acts like a drug. It's been established that it's even more addictive than cocaine.

Sugar releases pleasure hormones giving the brain an immediate high. We turn to chocolate or other sweet products when we're feeling down. Unfortunately, as with most stimulants, the high is only too brief, plunging us down into a low that makes the brain crave the pleasure again, and forces us to eat more sugar.

One effect of this is the well-known "sugar rush" phenomenon. This can affect anyone, but it's especially noticeable in children who consume many sweets and sugary drinks. It's no coincidence that the rise of hyperactivity in children is linked to high sugar intake.

How Does Sugar Affect Your Organs?

So far, you have learned that high sugar consumption can be harmful to your health. And in this section, you will look at how various organs in your body react to refined sugar.

How Does Your Pancreas React?

The pancreas produces insulin. When you consume too much sugar, and your body doesn't react to insulin effectively, your pancreas begins to pump out more insulin. Your pancreas will eventually fail, causing blood glucose levels to increase, putting you at a greater risk of heart failure and type 2 diabetes.

How Does Your Heart React?

When your diet includes too much sugar, the elevated insulin level in your system causes severe problems in the arteries throughout the whole body. It triggers inflammation in the arterial walls of your heart, making them thicker and stiffer, which has a detrimental impact and destroys heart health over time. It increases the risk of heart illnesses, such as strokes, heart attacks, and heart failure.

How Does Your Liver React?

High fructose corn syrup or fructose is abundantly found in added sugar. Fructose is processed in the liver and can cause liver damage if consumed excessively. Fructose is converted to fat in the liver after it is broken down. It can result in non-alcoholic steatohepatitis (NASH) and non-alcoholic fatty liver disease (NAFLD).

How Do Your Joints React?

Here's another reason to avoid excessive sugar if you suffer from joint pain. It has been discovered that sugar can worsen joint soreness because of the inflammation sugar triggers in the body. Sugar consumption has also been linked to a higher incidence of rheumatoid arthritis.

How Do Your Teeth React?

It is important to remember that high sugar consumption can lead to tooth decay. As mentioned previously, sugar affects your teeth badly. Here, streptococcus mutans bacteria eat any sugar left in your mouth and ferment it into lactic acid, causing the minerals found in tooth enamel to eventually dissolve.

How Does Your Skin React?

Another serious consequence of inflammation is that it may lead to skin ageing. The processed sugar binds to proteins in the blood, forming dangerous compounds known as advanced glycation end products (AGEs). These compounds age your skin. Protein fibres like elastin and collagen, which make your skin firm and young, eventually get damaged, leading to the skin becoming saggy and the appearance of wrinkles.

How Does Your Brain React?

Sugar causes your brain to release a high level of dopamine, a feel-good hormone, which explains why you may crave a sugary snack, especially when you're feeling down or stressed. Since healthy food such as fruits and vegetables don't trigger the brain to produce high amounts of dopamine, your brain begins to want sugar to experience similar satisfaction. On the other hand, too much sugar in foods can have a negative impact on your memory and attention.

How Do Your Kidneys React?

If you have diabetes, consuming excess sugar could harm your kidneys. The kidneys are responsible for purifying your blood. They begin to produce extra glucose into your urine once blood glucose levels reach a particular level. Diabetes, if left untreated, can harm the kidneys, preventing them from fulfilling their role of eliminating waste from the bloodstream. This could result in kidney failure.

My final thought in this section is that if you want to live a long and healthy life, you need to eliminate any refined sugar from your diet or minimise your consumption.

The next section will examine why people want to stop eating sugar. I want you to pay special attention to this part and start thinking of your own possible reasons for quitting sugar.

Time to Quit Eating Sugar

I have so far mentioned several health issues caused by consuming too much sugar. But abstract health warnings such as poor dental health, obesity, type 2 diabetes, or high blood sugar are still insufficient motivations for many people. The risk of various diseases is not taken seriously as most people tend to prioritise their well-being only after their health has been affected.

So far, we've looked at several negative effects sugar can bring to your health. Being aware of the positives as well as the negatives is equally important. We'll go into more detail about this later in the book.

Most of my clients want to stop consuming or reduce sugar from their diet because they want to increase their energy, look younger, or decrease their anxiety levels. You might have different motives. But looking after your health should be your main reason for quitting or reducing the consumption of sugary products. Making sure you don't overeat foods rich in sugar — whether you notice that your health is already suffering because of it or not — should be your *top* most *priority*.

I know that reducing or completely giving up on sugar can be extremely hard, especially if you experience intense cravings. Therefore, it is vital to understand why you want to quit, why it is important to you, and why now.

There is a wide range of motives and desires for people to change, and when it comes to quitting sugar, here are some of the most common reasons:

1. *You have a specific health issue*: Perhaps you've been diagnosed as pre-diabetic or warned you're at a higher risk of a heart attack. In which case, your well-being, and possibly your life, maybe tied in with a commitment to healthy eating and giving up sugar.
2. *You're overweight*: We know that being overweight is unhealthy, but it can also affect you in other ways. You might feel embarrassed wearing a bikini on the beach or be forced to give up activities you used to love (sports, dancing, etc.) because you're unfit or because it affects your confidence. If you know that cutting out sugar could significantly aid weight loss and help you reverse these issues, that's a powerful reason in itself.
3. *You're experiencing mood swings*: We'll look at this in greater detail later, but sugar can impact your mental and physical health, often causing mood swings. While these can have other causes, there is a chance that they could be brought on by being addicted to sugar.
4. *Sugar can make you look older*: Besides all the other damage it can do, sugar encourages the production of free radicals that cause the signs of ageing. Giving up sugar and replacing it with a healthy diet can give your body the chance to purge itself of the free radicals and repair some of the damage, particularly to the skin. This means that giving up sugar can help you look younger.
5. *Making menopausal symptoms worse*: Menopause and sugar don't go well together. Sugar can worsen menopausal symptoms and increase the frequency or the length of your hot flushes and night sweats.

Quitting eating sugar can reduce unpleasant symptoms and make you feel better.

6. *You experience sugar cravings*: Do you find it hard to get through the day without chocolate or cakes? Is it difficult to stop once you've started eating sweet foods? Is it unthinkable to have a meal without a sweet dessert? This is the effect of sugar addiction, where the brain demands the temporary high sugar gives it. Breaking an addiction and feeling free again is a great reason to give up sugar.

7. *You have a weak immune system*: If you constantly suffer from colds, flu, or similar diseases, sugar might be impairing your immune system. Think what life would be like if you weren't feeling unwell so often.

8. *Your dental health is poor*: If you need fillings or extractions regularly when you visit the dentist, it may be a sign that you are overeating sugar. Getting these procedures done may be unpleasant and expensive, which is an excellent reason to start focusing on healthy eating.

These eight reasons are the most common ones. They often motivate people to stop their bad eating habits. Can you relate to any of them?

You are at the end of Day One. It's time to do the task where you'll look deeply into your *why* and establish the primary motivation for giving up sugar. Understanding your *why* is crucial, so let's dig deep into it.

Day One Task: Identify Your Why

I've already mentioned plenty of important reasons for giving up sugar, but your particular motive could be different and more specific to you. It might include having a desire to fit into that dress again for a particular event, or you may want to improve your energy levels so you can play with your grandchildren and enjoy your life more, or maybe it's something else. Only you have the answer.

Giving up sugar will not be easy, and your determination to quit sugar will unlikely come from simply being told that it's unhealthy. The motivation that comes from within you is what will push you forward. That is a more powerful reason for changing your behaviour than hearing other people telling you what you should or shouldn't be doing.

I have prepared some questions to help you understand your circumstances and identify your *why*.

If you haven't done it already, please go to bit.ly/sugar-detox-workbook, and download the accompanying Workbook, *The 10 Day Sugar Detox Workbook*. The Workbook will support you in navigating through this book and give you extra tools to achieve your goal.

Most of the written exercises in the Workbook can also be found in this book, but for your convenience, I recommend downloading it as it'll help you keep all your answers in one place. In addition, you will find lots of valuable resources not included in this book. Your Workbook will be your go-to guide when you experience sugar cravings, are unsure what to eat, or simply want to remind yourself of your triggers.

Now, let's start with the first exercise.

Here are seven powerful statements, and I want you to fill out the blanks for each one of them:

1. I want to stop eating sugar because I want to be able to ACHIEVE....
2. I want to stop eating sugar because I want to LOOK....
3. I want to stop eating sugar because I want to FEEL....
4. I want to stop eating sugar because I want to EXPERIENCE....
5. I want to stop eating sugar because I want to HAVE....
6. I want to stop eating sugar because I want to BECOME....
7. I want to stop eating sugar because.... (choose something that speaks to you the most).

This exercise is designed to help you identify seven solid reasons that are personal only to you. Those reasons will motivate you to quit eating sugar and encourage you to maintain your goal.

When changing any behaviour, we need the motivation to help us begin the change, and we also need the motivation to stick to it. That's the reason why this written exercise is so powerful. It enables you to identify why you want to change and understand the reasons beyond the surface to continue your new healthy habit.

Now, have a look at your answers from the exercise that you just did and ask yourself the following questions:

- If I *can* achieve, look, feel, experience, have, or become what I want, how will my life or health improve?
- If I *can* achieve, look, feel, experience, have, or become what I want, how will my life or health be different?
- If I *can't* achieve, look, feel, experience, have, or become what I want, who will be affected and how?

Answers to these questions should give you your *why*. And when you're struggling to resist the temptation to reach for the chocolate bar or accept a delicious-looking cake, you can remind yourself of what you're doing, and WHY you're doing it.

Chapter 2

Day Two: All Sugar Isn't Bad

Welcome to Day Two!

Did you make it through yesterday without falling back on sugary foods? Today might be more challenging, but you can get through it and look forward to feeling like a new person in the long run.

Some people will have no problems when trying to remove sugar from their diet in the first couple of days, but others might experience some mild withdrawal symptoms.

Each person is different, and if you're doing this challenge with a friend or a family member, one of you may suffer from a slight headache, experience brain fog, or be ravenously hungry. Those symptoms are sometimes noticeable in some individuals on the second day of a sugar-free diet. But keep going, and ensure that you're eating substantial, well-balanced meals with plenty of protein and healthy fat (such as nuts or oily fish).

Today, I'll explain the different types of sugar — healthy and unhealthy — and discuss sugar addiction. You'll learn how sugar might be disguised in the ingredient lists of various foods. It might surprise or even shock you.

At the end of this chapter, you'll complete a task. Your task today will be to analyse your diet and identify where sugar is hiding in your food. This will be an essential stepping stone toward your sugar-free journey.

Different Types of Sugar

As previously explained, sugar is a naturally occurring soluble carbohydrate in most whole foods. However, it is not just one thing but an entire class of simple carbohydrates.

Sugars can be broadly divided into two types:

1. *Monosaccharides*: Consisting of individual sugar molecules.
2. *Disaccharides*: Consisting of two sugar molecules bound together, often but not always of different types.

The most common types of monosaccharides are:

- *Fructose*: Naturally occurring in fruit, some root vegetables and honey.
- *Glucose*: Naturally occurring in some fruit and vegetables. It is also formed from carbohydrates in the body.
- *Dextrose*: A variant of glucose, occurring naturally in grapes and other fruits, as well as honey.
- *Galactose*: It doesn't occur naturally in isolation but combines to form disaccharides.

The most common types of disaccharides are:

- *Lactose*: A combination of galactose and glucose, occurring naturally in milk and other dairy products.
- *Maltose*: Consisting of two glucose molecules found in various grains, especially barley.
- *Sucrose*: A combination of glucose and fructose, most commonly found in sugar cane and sugar beet, and is the type of sugar you're most likely to put in your tea or use in baking.

Monosaccharides and disaccharides are natural sugars and provide an essential part of a healthy diet. They're the primary source of glucose that plays a vital role in many of your body's functions. This type of sugar is "good sugar".

When the natural sources are processed to remove the sugar from the other parts of the plant, this forms free sugar, otherwise known as refined sugar. The most obvious example is when the sucrose is stripped from sugar cane or sugar beet and refined into granulated sugar or sugar cubes.

Free or refined sugar can cause various problems because your body relies on other nutrients from food, especially fibre, to break down the sugar when it enters the body. In free sugar, other nutrients have been removed.

Remember that if you're eating pure sugar, which was stripped from other nutrients (even when it's an ingredient in the recipe you are using), it can cause health issues.

How to Distinguish Between Different Types of Sugar

You have probably heard of simple and complex carbohydrates, but do you really understand the difference?

Here is a short description of each type: simple carbohydrates are formed of one or two sugar molecules, while the complex type is made of three or more sugar molecules. Due to different structures, they affect the body differently.

Simple carbohydrates, often known as processed sugar, are unhealthy. Looking at the food labels, you will notice that many foods have added sugar. Beware of this type of sugar. I have already explained the damaging effects on your health.

On the other hand, natural sugar can be found in fresh fruit and many vegetables, milk and dairy products, and grains. As long as no processing has taken place, these sources provide natural, healthy sugar.

However, sugar — particularly the simple type — can be hidden in various foods. Most packaged foods in boxes, jars, tins, cans, or plastic bags have likely been processed and contain added sugar.

In the next section of this book, you will learn that food labels often use a variety of names for sugar. Knowing the most common names will help you recognise them when reading food labels.

I'll explain how much sugar is in various foods later in the book, but the rule of thumb is that you can assume processed food contains free sugar. A great example would be fruit juice.

You might think that drinking unsweetened fruit juice is safe and sugar-free, but sadly it's often not the case. When you squeeze an orange, the processing strips away the other nutrients and turns them into free sugars, similar to sugar that you find in soda. When the natural sugar has been separated from the fibre and turned into free sugar, it is not as healthy as you thought it would be.

Similarly, you might assume that an unhealthy free sugar is a natural type: honey. What could be more natural than honey, you may ask? The problem is that it has already been processed by the bees and is almost pure sugar, without the balancing nutrients found in the plants it ultimately arrived from.

The Many Names for Sugar

Do you check the labels on the food you buy to see what it contains?

That's precisely what you should be doing. But unfortunately, it's not that simple. Sometimes labelling can be a minefield, and simply looking for the word "sugar" among the ingredients is often not enough. To truly understand where the sugar is hiding and that your diet is sugar-free, you need to learn various names for sugar.

I found over 80 words and phrases for the various types of sugar added to foods. Some may seem innocent enough, but you need to recognise that, as additives, these are all types of free or refined sugar.

Some sugar names include the word "sugar"; therefore, they

are easily identified as the foods we should reduce eating or avoid altogether. Some examples include demerara sugar, raw sugar, and yellow sugar. You may think they're healthier than "ordinary" sugar. But, even if there's a marginal difference, the fact remains that they're free sugars which means that consuming them in high doses could be detrimental to your health.

On the other hand, many names don't mention "sugar", and you may think they are natural products, but they are not.

The most common terms that don't mention sugar are:

- Agave nectar
- Barley malt
- Blackstrap molasses
- Brown rice syrup
- Buttered syrup
- Cane juice crystals
- Caramel Carob syrup
- Corn syrup
- Corn syrup solids
- Crystalline fructose
- Dextran
- Dextrose
- Diastatic malt
- Diastase
- D-ribose
- Ethyl maltol
- Evaporated cane juice
- Florida crystals
- Fructose
- Fruit juice
- Fruit juice concentrate

- Galactose
- Glucose
- Glucose solids
- Golden syrup
- High-fructose corn syrup
- Honey
- Isoglucose
- Lactose
- Malt
- Maltodextrin
- Maltol
- Malt syrup
- Maltose
- Mannose
- Maple syrup
- Molasses
- Muscovado
- Nectar
- Panela
- Panocha
- Refiner's syrup
- Rice syrup
- Saccharose
- Sorghum syrup
- Sucrose
- Sweet sorghum
- Treacle

You will find an even larger list containing the names for sugar in the Workbook. If you haven't downloaded it yet, it's time to do it now. Go to bit.ly/sugar-detox-workbook.

Please note that the food industry is constantly coming up with new euphemisms for sugar. If you don't recognise an item on an ingredient list, google it to find out what it is. Often, names we don't understand represent ingredients that can damage our health and should be avoided. Always choose items with fewer ingredients on the list.

What Makes Sugar so Addictive?

Sugar can be very addictive. This might seem like an extraordinary claim, but it's been established by scientific studies that rats and other animals can become physiologically dependent on sugar.[12] The research strongly suggests that this is likely to be the case in humans too.

This is because the glucose transmitted to the brain can stimulate the production of the neurotransmitter dopamine. Its role is to make us feel happy and positive. Dopamine stimulates the same emotional parts of the brain as drugs, such as cocaine, alcohol, nicotine, and opioids like heroin.

When the glucose is transmitted in quantities the brain requires, as it does when you stick to natural sugars, the effect is minimal. Refined sugars produce a significant amount of glucose, some of which end up unused in the brain. This will likely lead to a massive high — known as the "sugar rush".

However, as with all stimulants, the high is often followed by a corresponding low. Since the brain will have interpreted the high as a reward, it craves a repeat, and a signal will be sent that you need more of the food resulting in the high — chocolate, cakes or fizzy drinks, for instance.

This desire for more sugar will be partly conscious. After all, if eating something feels good, it's natural to want more of it.

The more dangerous impulses, however, are subconscious since they're harder to recognise and resist. You'll know that you want to have another of those delicious cakes. And then another, until you feel psychologically and emotionally satisfied. The need for sugar is rarely associated with physical hunger but with the desire to meet one or more of your emotional needs or get a quick energy boost.

Like any addictive substance, the more you give your brain this stimulus, the more it needs it. You'll sometimes feel extreme cravings to eat sugary foods and often binge on them. The high levels of refined sugar you're putting into your digestive system can weaken your metabolism and increase the risks of obesity, type 2 diabetes, heart disease, and various other illnesses and health conditions.

The trouble with bingeing on sugary foods is that, unlike someone taking heroin, most sugar addicts are blissfully unaware of their addiction. Many people talk about having a "sweet tooth" and how they can stop eating sugar any time they choose to — except that they don't have this choice.

I hope the task you completed yesterday helped you identify your *why*, and that your desire to give up sugar is more potent than before you started reading this book.

Today's task will help you look at your diet to identify where the sugar you eat is coming from.

Becoming aware of what you put in your body will help you be more in control of your eating habits and encourage you to make healthy sugar-free choices when planning your meals. As a result, you will be more energised, feel healthier, and have more confidence in your ability to give up sugar.

Day Two Task: Find the Sugar in Your Food

It is important to remember that there are both healthy and unhealthy sources of sugar.

Healthy sources include fresh fruit and vegetables (I recommend eating whole fruits instead of juicing them), unsweetened dairy products, and whole grains.

Most of the sweet foods you eat will contain added sugar, but you'll also find sugar in foods you wouldn't necessarily think contain sugar. This includes yoghurts, bread, breakfast cereals, many tinned fruit and vegetables, and some prepacked salads.

The various names for sugar should be included among the ingredients on the packets or tins, and the list of alternative names for sugar I've given you will help you to identify unhealthy products. As I've suggested, if you don't recognise an ingredient, get into the habit of looking it up.

I advise you to do the followings:

1. Look through your kitchen cupboards and fridge — or anywhere you keep food — look at the ingredient list on the back of each item and write down a list of every type of food you find that includes added sugar. If you're unsure about any item, add it to the list, anyway. It's better to be safe than sorry. Unless it's one of the healthy sources of natural sugar that I've already talked about, including these foods on the list would be the right choice.

2. Break down your list into sublists, depending on when you eat particular food: is it for breakfast? Chocolate would most likely be a snack. And if you eat a particular food more than once a day, then put it down as many times as you need to. Have a good look at your sublists. This exercise will give you a snapshot of where your unhealthy sugar comes from, how often you consume it, and what time of the day you're most likely to eat it.

3. Finally, write all the sugary foods that you consume, but don't keep in your home. This could include a spoon of sugar in your morning coffee that you have every morning while commuting to work or a few glasses of alcoholic drink after work.

Awareness will help you take control of your bad eating habits, enabling you to make healthier choices when planning and preparing meals. This will create a real difference in your health and well-being, giving your body what it requires instead of depriving it of its necessary nutrients.

If you haven't done it already, download the Workbook from bit.ly/sugar-detox-workbook, and go to Day Two. The instructions and the tables in the Workbook should make this process very easy to follow.

Chapter 3

Day Three: Identifying Sugar in Your Daily Life

Welcome to Day Three of the Sugar Detox Challenge!

How are you feeling today?

If you got used to eating lots of sugary foods, your body might respond to a lack of them in unusual ways on your third day of sugar detox. Your symptoms may remind you of a cold or flu, or you might even be experiencing fatigue.

There is no need to panic; you certainly don't need to contact your doctor about these symptoms. I can assure you that it's not uncommon for people to experience these symptoms on the third day of sugar withdrawal, but don't worry, as they will not last long.

I'd recommend you keep eating healthy meals and resist any instinct to reach for your everyday comfort foods — they're almost certainly loaded with sugar. And if you're physically very active, ensure you eat good carbs such as brown rice, whole-wheat pasta or potatoes. If you want something with a slightly sweet taste, try sweet potato as an alternative. Don't forget to balance your starchy meals with protein and healthy fats, and include a rainbow of fruit and vegetables.

Today, we'll continue to look at the sugar in your diet and identify where the sugar is lurking and in what quantities. You'll also learn how to avoid eating or drinking sugar, what sweeteners to avoid, and ways to sweeten your food in a healthy way.

Your task will be to identify which of your favourite foods have the most sugar because these will be the hardest to resist. On the other hand, if you learn that your favourite food has no added sugar, it can be a great way to maintain your sugar-free diet.

Where Can You Find Sugar and in What Amounts?

Yesterday, you found out about various sources of sugar in your food, but that doesn't explain how much sugar you're getting from them. So today, you're going to learn which types of food are the worst offenders.

Let me ask you this: "Have you ever tried to keep track of your sugar intake and given up because it's too confusing?" Yes, me too...before I discovered how to do it properly. At the time, I didn't understand the three things essential to make sense of sugar labelling on food packaging. They include:

- How do the various measurements (grams, teaspoons, calories) relate to one another?
- What portion sizes is sugar content measured by?
- How much sugar should I be eating daily?

Once I learned how to read the nutrition labels properly, it all started to make sense.

To answer the first question — one teaspoon of sugar is equivalent to 4g or 16 calories. There are three teaspoons in one tablespoon, which is equivalent to 12g of sugar and 48 calories.

The second question is considerably harder to answer since the servings on the packaging may not be the portion size that people usually go for. The best way to approach this would be to put together your typical portion of the food containing sugar and weigh it. For instance, pour out a bowlful of your favourite cereal, just as if you were going to have breakfast, and then tip it onto the scale.

You might find a significant difference between your portion size and the portion size on the packet, but you can easily calculate the amount of sugar in your portion from the information I have given you. For instance, if the packaging says that a serving of 40g contains 6.6g of sugar and you've found your food portions are 50% higher, this will give you a clear idea of how much sugar you consume. There'll be 8.25g in your food.

When reading labels, sugar will be usually listed under carbohydrates. Here's an example of what you may see on the nutrition label:

Nutrition Facts	
4 servings per container	
Serving size 1 bar (71g)	
Amount per serving	
Calorie 340	
	% Daily Value*
Total Fat 19g	**24%**
Saturated Fat 3g	**15%**
Trans Fat 0g	
Polyunsaturated Fat	2%
Monosaturated Fat	14%
Cholesterol 15mg	**5%**
Sodium 50g	**2%**
Total Carbohydrates	**10%**
Dietary Fibre 3g	**11%**
Total Sugars 19g	
Incl. 13g Added Sugars	**26%**
Protein 17g	**21%**

- Let's presume that your portion size is 2 bars. That means that you consume 26g of added sugar. This equals 6.5 teaspoons of sugar.

- It's important to remember that food containing more than 5 grams of sugar per 100g is the most urgent to cut out whether you are on a sugar-free diet or not.

- In this example, the serving size is 71g and has 13g added sugar, which means that 100g has approximately 18g added sugar, which is well above the recommended allowance.

The information on the packaging could be misleading. And if you don't know how to read nutrition labels properly, it's easy to get confused and overwhelmed.

As you can see from the example I've given you, the amount of sugar on the packaging shows "total sugars 19g, including 13g added sugars" per serving, which means that this product contains only 6g natural sugars.

When calculating the amount of sugar in your food, you need to consider your typical portion size. Looking at the above example, if your typical portion size is double the recommended amount, then you need to double the amount of sugar in your calculation. Sometimes, the nutrition label won't make it so obvious, and might only include the sugar amount in 100g of food. At other times, your portion size might not match the serving size written on the packaging. In this case, if you struggle to do the calculations — do some research. Just type "how much sugar is in a large bowl of, or in one small glass of (type the name)?", and you'll get the figure you are looking for.

To help you understand this better, I included some examples of several foods and drinks.

HOW MUCH SUGAR IS IN THE FOOD WE EAT				
Types of Food	Recommended Portion Size	Amount of Sugar	My Typical Portion Size	Amount of Sugar
Orange Juice	1 cup (248ml)	21g	2 cups (496ml)	42g
Nutella	2 tbs	21g	3 tbs	31.5g
Vanilla Ice Cream	½ cup	14g	1 cup	28g
Tomato Ketchup	1 tbs	3.7g	2 tbs	7.4g

As you can see from this example, the amount of sugar increased each time I increased the portion size.

What is the recommended maximum daily sugar intake, you may ask? This varies depending on your age and gender. A good set of figures to follow is this:

- Adult men: 36g (9 tsp or 3 tbs)
- Adult women: 24g (6 tsp or 2 tbs)
- Teens: 24-32g (6-8 tsp or 2-2.6 tbs)

Remember that these figures are the maximum safe levels. The less sugar you take, the better. And the more of this that can be replaced by natural sugar, the better.

So, where does the sugar you eat come from? It's a good question. Sugar is hiding in lots of foods, and the most common sources of added sugar include:

- Cakes and confectionery
- Sweets
- Desserts and ice-cream
- Chocolate
- Breakfast cereals
- Cereal bars
- Fruit in syrup
- Jam and marmalade
- Fast food
- Ketchup
- Alcohol
- Fizzy drinks
- Energy drinks
- Flavoured milk
- Various sauces

This is by no means an exhaustive list. You might be able to find sugar in foods that you'd never think of. It's safe to assume that any packaged or tinned food contains added sugar, even if it isn't sweet. For instance, a tin of Heinz tomato soup doesn't seem like a candidate for sweet food, does it? You might not realise that it contains nearly 20g of sugar per can — close to an adult woman's maximum daily intake in one go.

On the other hand, some are going to be no-brainers. An average bowl of Kellogg's Frosties contains 16g, while a packet of Sharwood's sweet & sour chicken (the clue's in the name) contains 24g. And how much Coke do you drink? Did you know that just one can of Coke can have 35g of added sugar?

These figures are frightening, and need to be considered when calculating your daily sugar intake. Remember that this doesn't apply to natural sugar that comes from whole foods. Let's look at the following example: An average-sized apple contains around 70% of the sugar quantity found in a Mars bar — but because it is made of natural sugar, there's no need to count it when calculating your daily intake.

I hope this section answered many questions about how much sugar you should be eating or how to calculate the amount of sugar in your favourite foods. But what happens if something you buy doesn't have packaging? We are going to look at this in the next section.

Ways You Unknowingly Eat Sugar

In the previous section, you learned how to check the nutrition information printed on the packaging and use it to calculate the amount of added sugar you're getting from the food it contains. But what if you cannot see the packaging of the foods and drinks you consume?

For example, if you buy a freshly baked loaf of bread. This contains just as much added sugar as a branded sliced loaf (around 3g per slice), but you'll have no way of finding that out.

So, what can you do?

Unless you know what to look out for, there are three sure ways of loading up with added sugar without any warning.

The first is alcohol — and, let's face it, most of us like a drink or two now and then, don't we? All alcoholic beverages contain some sugar, though the amount varies considerably. The stronger the alcoholic content, the lower the sugar content. Therefore, most spirits have low sugar content, while full-strength beers contain less sugar than light beers. Despite the amount of sugar in alcohol, there are many nutritional problems associated with it as well as the health and social dangers.

If you're a wine lover, you should know that wine does contain sugar, although the amount varies depending on the type. A standard glass of red wine has 0.91g of sugar, while white wine has 1.41g. Champagne, on the other hand, has 0.81g per glass.

However, these quantities are tiny compared to many cocktails, including sugar-laden soft drinks. While an ounce of Manhattan, for example, has 3g of sugar, one serving of Baileys contains 7.8g and Mojito 26g. To help you visualise this — Manhattan has just a little less than a spoon of sugar, Baileys has nearly two spoons, and Mojito has 6.5 spoons of sugar.

Another danger zone is likely to be your favourite takeaway. Chinese, Indian, Mexican — wherever it comes from, the chances are that there'll be plenty of added sugar in most of the dishes, along with other unhealthy additives like salt and MSG.

Similarly, you have very little chance of monitoring what's in your food when you're eating out. There's bound to be plenty of sugar if you go for fast food options, but it's unlikely you have any means of checking out the ingredients. If you have your heart set on a takeaway or a cocktail, you can look the sugar content up online and choose a lower-sugar option — and remember to count this into your daily sugar intake.

You will never know precisely what is hiding inside your food when eating out. Therefore, I always suggest to my clients to cook at home as often as possible or choose a restaurant with a more traditional menu. You'll be on much safer ground there.

Later in this book, I'll discuss how you can enjoy sugar-free eating out, but for now, let's look at how you might be consuming sugar unintentionally daily.

Avoiding Unintentional Sugar Consumption

When I seriously started looking at my sugar consumption and how I could reduce it, I estimated how much sugar I ate daily. The figure I came up with was disturbing enough — but when I revisited my figures a few months later, I realised that what I'd counted was barely a quarter of the actual figure.

It's very easy to underestimate how sugar builds up in a daily diet. Even though you are more familiar with the places where the sugar lurks than before you started reading this book, you might not know how much exactly it adds up to.

I want to give you an example of a typical day's eating by someone who isn't restricting their sugar intake. You will find that the amount of added sugar is astronomical. You'll discover that sugar is hiding in so many places, and the amount of sugar in most ordinary foods is vast.

Let's look at how much added sugar is in the typical diet of a person who doesn't pay attention to the amount of sugar they eat:

Breakfast:

- Glass of orange juice — 21g
- Coffee with one sugar — 4g
- One slice of white toast with butter and strawberry jam — 11g

Morning Snack:

- Coffee with one sugar — 4g
- Mars bar (standard) — 30.4g
- Bottle of Coke (370ml) — 39g

Lunch:

- Can of Heinz chicken & mushroom soup — 6.4g
- Weight Watchers summer fruit yoghurt — 6.1g

Late Afternoon Snack:

- Cup of hot chocolate — 24g

Dinner:

- Pizza — 10g
- Small slice of chocolate cake — 26g
- Glass of orange juice — 21g

That comes to a total daily sugar intake of 202.9g — well over five times the safe daily intake of added sugar for an adult man and more than eight times the level for an adult woman.

I want to remind you that there are four grams of sugar in one teaspoon. In this example, this person consumed just over 50 spoons of sugar in only one day.

You wouldn't deliberately take 50 spoons of sugar in a day, would you?

This is a great example explaining how by simply eating and drinking "normally", you can load yourself up with an unhealthy level of added sugar.

You have probably noticed that this person didn't overeat or binge. To most people, this is a normal way of eating. This suggests that most peoples' diets are very unhealthy and likely to contribute to obesity, heart disease and type 2 diabetes, among other conditions, not to mention being addicted to a substance that can send your moods careering from hyperactivity to a depressed state.

I hope that information I'm sharing with you in this book is helping you to recognise how much sugar is hiding in your food and motivates you to continue with the rest of the 10 Day sugar detox, leaving your sugar habits behind for good.

Healthy Substitutes and Alternatives for Sugar

So, you know that you need to avoid eating free sugar, but maybe you have a "sweet tooth", and your cravings are intense.

My clients often ask me whether I'd recommend using artificial sweeteners, either by adding them to the foods or drinks themselves, or by having them already been added.

Unfortunately, some artificial sweeteners can be more damaging to our health than using sugar. For example, sorbitol and other sugar alcohols used as artificial sweeteners are known to feed harmful bacteria in the large intestine. At the same time, aspartame and acesulfame-K have been linked to an increased cancer risk.

As shown by an analysis of the Harvard School of Public Health (HSPH) research, studies have suggested that many artificial sweeteners are linked to weight gain and increased blood sugar.[13] However, the review notes that more study is needed on the subject.

HSPH raises the issue of using artificial sweeteners to wean people off sugar in the short-term but questions how effective this would be. Since they don't give the brain the "reward" that sugar does, artificial sweeteners' effectiveness in reducing sugar dependence is likely to be limited.

In addition, it has been shown that many artificial sweeteners act in the same way as refined sugar by raising the glucose level in the blood. This increases the risk of putting on weight, cardiac disease and other health conditions.

So, where does this leave the use of artificial sweeteners, you may ask? According to studies, many sweeteners are associated with bad health, but others may not be healthier than using sugar — and they won't necessarily stop your sugar cravings.

That doesn't mean that you have to avoid anything that tastes sweet. As you know now, natural, healthy sugar occurs in many unprocessed foods, such as fruit and vegetables, and as long as you eat the whole food, your body should deal with the sugar without causing any harm to your health.

If you need to add sweetness to a recipe, there are natural alternatives to refined sugar or artificial sweeteners. I often add apple sauce or mashed banana to recipes, for instance, if I want to enjoy a little sweetness. And instead of adding sugar or honey to cereal, I recommend having some blueberries or other fresh fruit.

You don't even have to add anything sweet to satisfy your sweet tooth. Occasionally, adding a pinch of salt to a recipe can bring out the sweetness. Of course, like sugar, salt is another food that many of us overuse, but an odd pinch shouldn't be a problem if you're eating a healthy, natural diet. To be safe, use one of the more beneficial forms, such as sea salt.

Day Three Task: Find Out Which of Your Favourite Foods Have the Most Sugar

You went through the fridge and kitchen cupboards yesterday to determine which foods contain added sugar. And today, you'll examine which foods are the worst offenders.

To do this, you need to do the following. Go to the Workbook, and under Day Three, there is a section to write your answers.

Your task is to do the following:

1. Think about your favourite foods — ones you often feel a craving for, and do some brainstorming.
2. Choose five foods from the above list and add them to the table provided in the Workbook.
3. Make sure you read food labels carefully for all five items on your list of favourites. Go through them one by one and identify the foods with over 5g of sugar per 100g. No amount of sugar is healthy, and as I've mentioned before, foods with a large amount of sugar can be damaging to your health and should be avoided, whether you are following a sugar-free diet or not.
4. To find out the exact amount of sugar in the typical portion size of your favourite foods, use the example shown in the table, *How Much Sugar is in the Food We Eat*. This will help you better understand how much sugar you consume from each portion.

See you tomorrow for Day Four.

Chapter 4

Day Four: Removing Sugar From Your Diet

Welcome to Day Four!

I hope the headaches, brain fog, and cold-like symptoms you may have been suffering from due to sugar withdrawal are clearing up. And if you have started to experience mood swings due to a sugar-free diet, you will likely find everyone unusually irritating. The chances are that it's down to your mood rather than their behaviour, so make an effort to think before you snap.

You may also notice that you suffer from skin irritation or acne. Don't panic about it — it's just your body's way of cleaning out the toxins from your system, and your skin should start improving in a few days.

If you're not experiencing any of the symptoms I mentioned, consider yourself lucky. Not everyone will be affected in the same way.

Today, we'll be focusing on creating a healthy and balanced diet. It is all about learning to prepare healthy meals, becoming conscious of sugar in your drinks, and knowing what to pay attention to when shopping for sugar-free foods. And in addition to eating healthily, try taking milk thistle and ginger tea. They should help you with the detoxification process and support your overall well-being.

Today's task will continue to help you identify sugar in the food you buy, including paying attention to those eighty-plus alternative names for sugar.

What is a Healthy Diet?

So what is the best way of having a healthy diet?

Some people believe that eating one particular healthy food and consuming only that for breakfast, lunch, and dinner can provide the body with everything it needs. But, this is far from the truth.

Unfortunately, the healthiest food isn't going to be good for you if that's the only food you'll ever eat. Your body needs a variety of nutrients. Not a single food can provide your body with absolutely everything it needs. It is vital to follow a balanced diet and ensure that the nutrients you consume are from healthy sources and include a mix of micronutrients and macronutrients.

The primary nutrients you need to incorporate in your everyday diet include proteins, carbohydrates and fats (yes, fat can be healthy), as well as the range of vitamins and trace minerals you get from your "five a day". In most cases, there are healthy and unhealthy ways of getting these nutrients into your body.

The exact proportion of the "macronutrients" (proteins, carbohydrates and fats) will vary slightly depending on various factors such as climate and lifestyle. However, for a typical person in most developed countries, the suggested proportions of your daily calorie intake are:

- *Proteins*: 15% or a little more
- *Carbohydrates*: There are many different types, but ideally, a little below 60%
- *Fats*: 20-35%, as long as it's a healthy fat[14]

However, there are many variables, but these figures should be seen as starting points for designing your healthy diet.

Another critical piece of advice I can give you is to include healthy sources of these macronutrients. As you now know, sugar is a carbohydrate, and you certainly don't want your daily allowance of carbs to consist of refined sugar.

More detailed information about a healthy diet can be found in two of my books *Get Healthy on a Tight Schedule* and *Get Fit and Healthy in Your Own Home in 20 Minutes or Less*. But I'll summarise the basics of a healthy diet here.

Protein

It is found in meat, fish and dairy, but these aren't the only sources of protein. If you eat meat, try to eat lean cuts if possible. They contain fewer calories and fats. And if you're a vegetarian or vegan, you can get your protein from soy, nuts, and beans. These will be your primary protein sources.

Carbohydrates

They are divided into starch, fibre and sugar. Natural, healthy sugars are mainly found in fresh fruit, vegetables, and dairy products. Starch comes primarily from potatoes, bread, rice, pasta, and cereals. Always choose whole grains as they are a healthier option. Potatoes should be boiled instead of fried or baked, preferably with their skins still on. Potato skins are good sources of fibre, as well as pulses, legumes, fruit and vegetables.

Fats

This macronutrient comes in several varieties. It is the saturated and trans fats that are bad for your health as they can increase the risks of obesity and heart disease. Unsaturated fats such as olive oil, avocados, nuts, and oily fish play a vital role in keeping your body healthy, as long as you don't overeat them.

Many people eat too many nuts once they learn they are good for them. But remember, overeating any type of food is not good for you, even if it's healthy.

Besides macronutrients, your body also needs vitamins and minerals. They are called micronutrients.

Vitamins

They are found mainly in fresh fruit and vegetables, and the best advice to give you is to "eat the rainbow". This is because the colour reflects the specific nutrients that the food is rich in. Therefore, consuming the rainbow of different colours from natural foods will ensure that your body gets what it needs.

Essential *Minerals*

These can be found in most healthy foods, but make sure you're not cutting them out if you follow a specific diet. For example, red meat is a rich source of iron, but if you're a vegetarian, you need to look for other foods rich in iron, such as broccoli or spinach.

Learning to Prepare Sugar-Free Meals

So far, it is hopefully becoming clearer which types of foods to include and avoid when following a sugar-free diet.

It is very easy to consume a high amount of sugar unknowingly due to confusing food labels, but once you learn how to read them and how to identify sugar from the lengthy ingredient list, you'll be able to remove sugary products from your surrounding.

This section will teach you how to put a few healthy ingredients together and create sugar-free meals.

Here is a range of options you might consider for your sugar-free (and otherwise healthy) meals. The exact content will vary according to your taste.

- *Breakfast*: Great options include overnight oats, scrambled, boiled egg, or omelette. Various vegetables such as mushrooms, peppers and onions. They can be added to an egg omelette. Fresh fruits such as a medium-sized apple with a few nuts, or spoons of Greek yoghurt with berries and sprinkled seeds on top, are an excellent idea to start the day. You can also eat them as a snack later in the day.

- *Lunch and dinner*: Some great sugar-free suggestions include grilled chicken and other lean meat, oily fish or a soya substitute, salad, and roasted or boiled vegetables — make sure you have as many colours as possible. Think of the rainbow.
- *Snacks:* Fresh fruit and nuts are ideal if you need to snack between meals. Alternatively, you may choose to snack on vegetable sticks. They are a great alternative.
- *Drinks*: Drink plenty of water throughout the day. And if you want to add a bit of flavour, add a slice of citrus fruit to your filtered glass or a water bottle. If you want a hot drink, unsweetened herbal teas are the best.

These suggestions are by no means the only options. As you get used to sugar-free eating and better at identifying which foods are safe to eat, you can become creative and start experimenting. You'll find that, far from being restrictive, a sugar-free diet offers endless opportunities. The best way to think about it is that it includes most, if not all-natural foods. All-natural excludes all processed foods with added sugar. There are plenty of foods you can consume, all bursting with healthy nutrients.

You can see from the example I gave you that a sugar-free diet is relatively easy to plan. You just need to include plenty of protein, healthy fats and complex carbohydrates. These micronutrients play different but essential roles in the body taking care of your overall health and well-being.

Later in the book, you will find 30 anti-inflammatory recipes to give you plenty of ideas and help you plan your sugar-free diet.

But now, let's learn how to make sugar-free desserts. It's easier than you think.

Making Sugarless Desserts

When you decided to start on this programme to give up sugar, you probably assumed that you would have to say goodbye to desserts.

So, how can you have a sugar-free dessert?

Perhaps the most obvious choice would be to make a fresh fruit salad. But there are many more choices than that. Here are a few suggestions to illustrate the range of options you can have:

- If you have an ice cream maker, you can make it exactly as you usually would, using milk, cream, egg yolks and vanilla, but sweetening it with fresh fruit instead of artificial sweetener.
- Fruit crumble is usually packed with sugar, but there's no reason why it has to be. If you include naturally sweeter fruits like strawberries, you'll have a tarter crumble than usual, but it can still taste delicious. You can top it with natural yoghurt.
- Carrot cake is a relatively healthy form of cake, but it traditionally contains sugar in the cake and the icing. However, it will still taste delicious if you simply leave the sugar out and use almond flour instead of white flour.
- How about mango and lime mousse for your dessert?

This can be made from gelatine, fresh mangos, lime zest, double cream, and no added sugar.

These are just a handful of the options you have for delicious sugar-free desserts. For example, you can enjoy desserts just as much on your sugar-free diet as you did before. You'll find plenty of recipes online — but you need to be cautious.

Some recipes you'll find interpret honey or maple syrup as "sugar-free" alternatives. Do you remember the list of sugars in Chapter Two? You'll know that these are just some of the many names for sugar.

Similarly, these recipes often remove the sugar by using artificial sweeteners. As I explained in Chapter Three, though, many artificial sweeteners act much the same way as refined sugar, and some have an even higher health risk.

Another thing to look out for in recipes is when you're told to use a ready-made ingredient. This is probably fine in most cases, but there's no guarantee they won't contain sugar. The best advice is to treat these like any other food — check the ingredients listed on the packaging to be sure that the item is sugar-free.

However, as long as you take precautions, you can enjoy delicious desserts that contain no sugars other than the natural ones in fruit or dairy products.

Stop Drinking Sugar

Most people are aware that certain types of foods contain lots of sugar, but they are less aware of the sugar in their drinks.

So far in this book, I have already mentioned some drinks containing free sugars even though they are described as "unsweetened". This is particularly true for fruit juices, whether that's orange juice, pineapple juice or mixed tropical fruits.

The manufacturers portray these drinks as healthy, but turning them from whole fruits to isolated juice also turns their natural sugars into free sugars. For example, in Tropicana mango juice, there is 30g of free sugar per 200ml, representing a medium-sized glass. Many other soft drinks, whether sweetened fruit squashes or fizzy drinks contain even more sugar.

I have already mentioned Coca-Cola several times in this book, and you have previously learnt that there's 35g of sugar in one can of Coke. Energy drinks are even higher in added sugar, so I strongly recommend avoiding them.

And what about sports drinks? Did you know that some sports drinks can have more than 48g of sugar in a bottle, that's over 12 teaspoons of sugar?

Your favourite hot drink might not be much better. A Costa Massimo Caramel latte will deliver 35g of sugar, a Starbucks hot chocolate 34g, and a Yazoo strawberry milkshake 46g. Just one of these drinks a day will take you into dangerous territory.

I explained on Day Three that all alcoholic drinks contain some sugar, though the amount varies widely. Although they aren't entirely sugar-free, stronger beers and pure spirits are the safest bets, while some cocktails are the worst offenders.

Remember that too much alcohol can damage your health in other ways, even if it isn't a significant sugar threat. So, pay careful attention to your alcohol intake.

The safest drink to stick to is filtered water. You can add a slice of fresh fruit to it if you prefer a bit of flavour. Milk is fine to drink in moderation, while unsweetened herbal teas are the best type of hot drink.

Other hot drinks that are sugar-free, natural, and healthy include adding ginger, a fresh slice of lemon, or fresh peppermint leaves to the hot water. Hot drinks that should be avoided include mocha, hot chocolate, Horlicks and Ovaltine, among many others. Ovaltine, a popular bedtime drink, contains 49g of sugar per 100g and 9g per serving which is one cup. That is more than two spoons of sugar, just before going to sleep.

How to Shop for Sugar-Free Foods

Is buying sugar-free foods straightforward?

When people start learning about sugar and find out that it is hiding in so many foods, the confusion often kicks in and shopping for sugar-free foods becomes a real struggle.

So what's the answer, you may ask?

Let's look at the most common struggles you may experience in this area. They are most likely to include the following:

I don't know where to look for sugar-free foods: Walking into a large food store and being surrounded by thousands of products could be overwhelming. Not many people know that most supermarkets have a similar layout, where within the first few aisles, you can find the freshest foods, like fruit, vegetables, meat, and dairy products. On the other hand, the further you go, the food becomes noticeably more unhealthy. The centre aisles are often filled with "junk" food and other ultra-processed foods high in salt, sugar, and fat. This might not apply to some smaller shops, but most larger stores have a similar landscape and understanding this can help you with your sugar-free shopping.

I don't understand food labels: This is a common problem. Many people struggle to understand how to decode food labels. I'll be talking about how to read labels later in the chapter, but for now, remember that it is essential to be prepared to read labels when doing food shopping, as that's the only way to discover the hidden places for sugar. I suggest you always take the list of alternative names for sugar I gave you on Day Two. As I've mentioned already, you will find a more extensive list of names for sugar in the Workbook, and if you haven't downloaded it already, it's time to download it now. Go to bit.ly/sugar-detox-workbook, and you'll find the list called *Many Names for Sugar* on Day Three.

I cannot resist various foods displayed on the supermarkets' shelves: How many times have you walked into a shop, looked around and seen colourful designs on food packaging calling your name? You couldn't resist the temptation, and within a few short minutes, you've started to fill your trolley with various packets and tins of foods containing sugar, additives and preservatives to look and taste good, and last longer. One way to solve this problem is to never do grocery shopping on an empty stomach.

I never know what to buy, so I always need to look around the shop: Sometimes we don't know what to buy for tomorrow's dinner or Sunday's lunch, so we walk up and down the aisles, checking the packaging of various products. I suggest you plan meals for the week and create a shopping list based on your plan.

Here is a tip: Do not do the menu plan when you are hungry. The best time to do it is when you are feeling full such as after eating dinner. This is the time when you are least likely to crave unhealthy foods. Going to the shop with your list and sticking to it as much as possible will help you resist the temptation to go after all those "amazing special offers" and colourful boxes of packaged foods.

These are a few ideas to make your sugar-free shopping easier to deal with and help you to stick to a sugar-free diet.

Try to think of your sugar-free shopping as a treasure hunt, where every healthy food you add to your cart is a treasure — a reward that brings you closer to your goal. This will give you a sense of adventure and an open mind — a "can-do" attitude.

Ways Sugar Can Sneak Into Your Shopping Trolley

It isn't easy to identify sugar in your food. Who'd suspect something as innocent as unsweetened fruit juice to contain large quantities of sugar?

I've mentioned reading labels several times, but there are two significant problems with this. The ingredients list often includes items you might not recognise, and the other is that the quantities are sometimes misleading.

On Day Two, I explained the many names for sugar and how some of these may give a false impression that they are actually good for you. For instance, they may include types of sugar like fructose or lactose, which are often associated with being healthy, natural sugars. However, if they're listed as ingredients, they're free sugars.

In addition, some of the names seem almost to have been designed to be perceived as being attractive and healthy. Terms like agave nectar and barley malt sound very natural, but they still contain sugars. Similarly, even words that mention sugar can convey a healthier impression. Raw sugar, for instance, sounds like it's natural and back-to-basics — but this is also simply added sugar and doesn't have more nutritional value than white or brown sugar.

Some phrasing can be misleading. For example, a can of baked beans contains a considerable amount of sugar. Some brands offer a "reduced salt and sugar" version, and you may assume they are a healthy version. In fact, there's a big difference between "reduced sugar" and "sugar-free". You'll need to determine how much sugar these contain in the-long term and calculate whether it's negligible enough for an occasional treat. For the time being, while you're detoxing from sugar, it's best to avoid these foods.

Besides misleading claims, some items you might want to buy, such as freshly baked bread, may not have any labelling on them. Unless it belongs to one of the safe categories, such as fresh and unmodified fruit, vegetables, meat, fish, dairy etc., make sure you research it before buying. If necessary, get your phone out and google it. You'll be protecting your health.

Day Four Task: Take a Shopping Trip

As you come towards the end of Day Four of going sugar-free, your task is to take a shopping trip where you will read the nutrition labels and identify the foods loaded with sugar and those that are safe to eat. This might not be your typical shopping day, but it'll be the beginning of replacing some of your old unhealthy shopping habits with new ones that will benefit your health.

First, make a shopping list. This task includes making your list similar to what you normally would buy.

It is important to follow the instructions provided in the Workbook. You will find a table divided into two parts — unsafe and safe. You will need to decide where to allocate the items from your shopping list. Items belonging to the safe groups would include lemons, smoked salmon, onions, etc. The items belonging to the unsafe group would be fruit juice and sweet popcorn.

If you are in doubt and unsure which list a particular item belongs to, include it in the unsafe group.

Then, you'll need to find healthy alternatives to the items in your unsafe group and write them in the safe group. The example is shown in the Workbook.

You should have two safe groups now. Copy items from each group in the space provided in the Workbook.

You are now ready for your shopping trip.

When you arrive at the store, give yourself plenty of time. You'll be checking the labels of all items on the *safe* list you created. There are two main things you'll be looking at on each packaged food:

1. Read carefully through the list of ingredients. Put the item back on the shelf if you notice any of the alternative names for sugar on the list. Think about other ingredients too, and ask yourself whether they could be a source of free sugar — e.g. if syrup is listed.
2. Check the nutritional information, noting the sugar quantity per serving and the serving size. Even if the sugar appears to be natural, a high level in a serving means that the item is best avoided, at the very least, while you're detoxing from added sugar. If an item is unsuitable, look for a healthier alternative. And if you can't find a healthier option to replace it with, I suggest you leave it on the shelf and do the research when you get home to get ideas for the replacement.

After the shopping trip, I suggest that you go to the Workbook and note down what you've learned — write a list, draw a chart, etc., whatever helps you best support your learning and develop new healthy habits.

Make a conscious decision to consume only healthy alternatives for the rest of your detox.

Writing a shopping list, splitting it into safe and unsafe parts, and reading nutrition labels might seem overwhelming for you at this stage. But don't worry, this will become easier once you adopt this behaviour as a part of your routine.

Behaviour that is repeated numerous times will eventually turn into a habit. And when this happens, you will do things on autopilot, and you won't need to write lists or keep notes unless you want to. You will make a mental note of what you want to do or need to do, and your habits will lead the way.

When you develop a habit of eating a healthy, balanced diet, you will notice changes in how you look and feel. This will encourage you to continue with a new way of eating, and in no time, you will accept your sugar-free diet as a welcome change in your life.

Chapter 5

Day Five: Removing Sugar from Your Surroundings

Welcome to Day Five!

By Day Five of your sugar detox, if you were experiencing headaches over the last few days, they should be gone by now, and the cravings you've been feeling for sugary foods should be more manageable. That doesn't mean that the struggle is over, but resisting the temptation is likely to be easier.

Today, we'll look at how you can remove the sugar from your environment so that it's not constantly tempting you. I'll explain how to identify sugar in your surroundings and why being surrounded by sugar can lead to failure. You'll also learn how to sugar-proof your home and office and look at some sugar-free meals.

Identify Sugar in Your Surroundings

In the western world, most households are loaded with sugar. And if you share the house with other family members or housemates, and they don't follow the same diet as you, I strongly suggest you go through your fridge or kitchen cupboards.

You already did the first part of this exercise at the end of Day Two of this challenge, but today, I'm asking you to repeat the process, take action, and clear your environment of sugar.

When going through the kitchen, be thorough — check nutrition labels on all condiments as they often contain added sugar. And if you find tomato ketchup, salad cream, or mayonnaise, you'll need to stay well clear of them as they are sugar-rich foods.

Here is a list of some most common foods containing sugar that you'd never think of them that way. They include the following:

- Bread
- Flavoured yoghurt
- Breakfast cereals
- Instant oatmeal
- Nut butter
- Granola bars
- Bottled flavoured water
- Bottled tea
- Protein powder
- Most sauces
- Energy bars

At first glance, some of these foods seem to be harmless when it comes to sugar content. But remember — unless the food is natural and hasn't been processed, you won't be wrong in assuming it contains some processed sugar.

Most packaged foods are loaded with sugar. It is your responsibility to learn where sugar is, which form it commonly occurs in, and familiarise yourself with various names the food industry uses to hide sugar in the foods.

Let me make one thing clear. You're always in control of what you put inside your body. And yes, food manufacturers add lots of free sugar to our foods, and marketers are trying to hide the truth from us with clever marketing messages that often sound confusing. My advice is, if you're offered something from a packet, tin, can, bag or box, politely refuse it, and if you see it in the shop, make sure you read the nutrition label, or simply put it back on the shelf.

It might also be a good idea to research the product afterwards, in case you come across it again in the future. Your knowledge about certain foods will help you to respond with more confidence next time.

I remember when I started following a gluten-free and dairy-free diet. I was confused about which foods contained gluten or milk. After doing my own research, I gained plenty of confidence to make the right decision about whether I wanted to eat a certain food or not.

Doing your own research and getting familiar with food labels on food packaging is crucial. It will help you judge which foods are sugar-free and which are not and which are safe to eat and which are not.

Don't allow the food industry to control you. Make sure you are in control.

How Having Sugar Around You Leads to Failure

We have all been there. A plate of cakes someone thoughtfully provides for you when you visit them, sitting in the middle of the table calling your name, and you tell yourself, "One slice won't hurt." Or you walked down the aisle in your local store surrounded by cookies, chocolate bars, etc., and you say, "I'll start my diet tomorrow." Does this sound too familiar?

You are right, one piece of cake won't hurt, and you can always start your diet tomorrow, but how many times have you said this?

Do you understand why this is happening and why your desire for sugar is so strong?

It happens because sugar is highly addictive. Just like someone who's previously been addicted to alcohol or nicotine, when sugary foods are right there in front of you, they cause temptation. You're tempted not because you're weak, but because you remember how great it is to get that sugar rush. You felt a sudden burst of energy that made you feel happy for a while.

What happens straight afterwards is called a sugar crash. It is the opposite of feeling happy and high. A sugar crash is a sudden drop in blood sugar levels that can cause anxiety and hunger, and make you feel shaky and irritable.

"Is it possible to stop cravings for sugary foods?" I often hear this question.

It's certainly possible to resist sugar cravings. After living sugar-free for a while and your body has been thoroughly detoxed, your taste has changed. You'll no longer be craving sugar. Remember, your body cannot crave foods you don't eat; you can only crave the taste and texture of foods you are familiar with. In other words, you can only crave foods that you consume regularly. That's why the 10 Day sugar-free detox challenge is a great way to stop your sugar addiction. After 10 days of following a sugar-free diet, your cravings will subside, your body will feel healthier, you will have more energy, and no more foggy brain — you will think clearer.

After working with so many clients over the years, helping them improve their diet and beat their sugar addiction, I noticed that the need to eat sugar is not only caused by the need to provide them with more energy or satisfy their physical hunger. Sometimes it is used as a strategy to deal with discomfort and unhappy emotions, or it's simply a habit.

At the initial stage of this process, when you are still working on developing your sugar-free lifestyle, it is important to make sure you aren't being constantly exposed to the temptation of sugary food and drinks. While you may be fine treating yourself to something sugary on a special occasion when the sugar-free diet becomes a part of your life, at this stage, a relapse could undo days or even weeks of good work.

Not only could this start up the vicious cycle of highs, lows and cravings, but it can do a lot of damage to your morale and motivation. You may feel like a failure, and find it hard to get back on track and continue the detox.

Ensuring that your surroundings are sugar-free as much as possible at this stage of the process is crucial. You may be able to resist buying a cake or a bar of chocolate while shopping and walking down the aisle, but if you know that there are sugary foods in your home or place of work, it could be difficult to constantly fight the urges, so you'll be more likely to give in to them.

This makes it vital that you sugar-proof your home and workplace, at least until you are fully confident in your ability to resist that voice. But how do you go about that, when other people may still be bringing sugary foods into your zone?

We'll discuss this in the next section.

How to Live with Your Friends, Family, and Sugar

How often have you been out with friends when someone holds a bag of snacks and says, "Do you want one?" and you can't say no? Yes, so have I. After all, it would be rude not to accept, wouldn't it?

Unfortunately, unless the friend is experienced in sugar-free eating, those snacks are probably loaded with sugar — even if they don't seem to be obviously sweet.

Let's take a look at crisps as an example. They're salty rather than sweet, but that doesn't make them sugar-free. Amounts vary considerably. For example, Walkers cheese & onion crisps contain 0.8g of sugar per 25g. That might not seem too bad, but it's 0.8g too much. In any case, like many other types of snacks, crisps are designed to make you keep reaching for more. I used to work with a client who, before we started working together, used to have between four to six bags of crisps one after another.

Many similar snacks, such as Kettle Vegetable Chips, have even more sugar in them. The name of the snack might sound like there is healthy food in the bag, but it contains over 21g of sugar per 100g. While some of it may have come from the various vegetables that flavour them, this does not make them healthy — they contain free sugar.

You need to be extra cautious in social situations. Accepting foods from friends, particularly snacks, is one of the ways sugar can ambush you.

It would be ideal, of course, if everyone in your household joined you in going sugar-free, but if this is not the case, you need to be aware of the ever-present temptation. People you live with might be bringing food home loaded with sugar, as they are unaware of the sugar content.

Remember, there's a higher percentage of foods containing sugar, than foods that don't have any sugar. Therefore, there is a high possibility that the food someone offers you or brings home will contain some kind of sugar.

If your loved ones are not on the same journey as you, the best thing you can do is to talk to them — explain how important it is for you to give up sugar. Make it clear that you're not trying to force them to join you, but ask them to respect your position. Perhaps you could arrange to keep your food and theirs separately. It will make it easier for you to avoid temptation.

If they are open to improving their health, consider educating them. That is the best thing you can do for someone you love and care about. Share the knowledge you are gaining from this book and ask them to join you on your sugar-free journey. And when they start noticing positive changes in their health, experience more energy, have younger-looking skin, lose weight, and the chances of developing life-threatening conditions such as cardiovascular disease have decreased, they'll be thankful to you.

Involving the whole family in following the sugar-free diet and committing to making better dietary and lifestyle changes is the best thing you can do for the people you love.

How to Sugar-Proof Your Home and Workplace

At the most basic level, you already know how to sugar-proof your environment. The tasks you've completed so far at the end of each chapter have helped you identify which foods and drinks in your home contain added sugar.

If you live by yourself, going through the cupboards and fridge, armed with the lists you have made, and getting rid of anything you have marked as containing added sugar, should be a relatively easy task. After doing so, you have a few choices: Any food containing sugar can be thrown in the bin, donated to a food bank, or offered to a friend who is happy to accept it.

I understand that doing this exercise is probably easier said than done, as most likely you'll be getting rid of many of your favourite foods, but that's the sugar addiction talking. You need to be ruthless.

I remember when I first made the decision to go sugar-free, how hard it was to get rid of those chocolate biscuits, sugary cereals and flavoured yoghurts.

Communication is key.

It is important to communicate with people close to you about your intentions, what you are trying to achieve, and why you are doing it. Otherwise, doing this task could be even more challenging. Asking for support indicates bravery and should not be seen as a sign of weakness.

Speak to people in your household about why you want to give up on eating sugar and find a way to keep your food separately, giving yourself a constant reminder that the sugary food isn't yours. Or even better, invite them to join you.

Having a shared workplace with several other people and keeping it sugar-free might seem even more difficult than sharing a house.

You might not be able to completely sugar-proof your working environment, but there is a lot you can do. Clearing your personal area could be an option. And if there's a shared kitchen, perhaps you could explain your situation to your colleagues and negotiate so you can have a sugar-free corner of the storage space where you can stock up with your healthy alternatives.

The harmful foods might still be there, but at least they won't be yours. And you never know — some of your colleagues might end up deciding to join you in your sugar-free corner.

As I've said earlier, the best thing is, once again, to talk to your colleagues and explain how important giving up sugar is to you.

After clearing your kitchen or your workplace from sugar-rich foods, you need to refill your empty fridge and kitchen cupboards with sugar-free alternatives. It's not enough to get rid of the wrong foods. You must have the right items available. Otherwise, you might reach for the wrong types of food when hunger strikes.

If you completed yesterday's task and did the shopping trip, that's great. I hope that following the lists of food that are safe and unsafe to eat, and checking nutrition labels on various items was not too overwhelming for you. And if you haven't done it yet, I suggest you do it before carrying on with today's task, where you will be removing sugary foods from your environment.

Day Five Task: Get Rid of Sugar From Your Home and Workplace

As you come to the end of Day Five of your sugar detox, hopefully, you're feeling a lot better and more positive.

You should definitely have turned the corner by now, and whatever symptoms you've been suffering from, you can expect them to start subsiding from now on.

The most important thing is to keep your focus and carry on eating healthily.

Your task for today is to clear your house of all the foods containing added sugar, making more space for the healthy foods that are either sugar-free or contain only healthy, natural sugars in their original context.

Follow these four steps:

1. Decide where you will put the food items you're getting rid of. A large, sturdy box would be ideal. Also, decide what to do with it once it gets full.
2. Check for the food around the house — your fridge, freezer, pantry, kitchen cupboards and any storeroom you may have away from the kitchen. Remove every item that has added sugar and place it in the box.
3. If you're unsure whether an item contains sugar or not, don't just ignore it. I suggest you read through the ingredient list on the back of the item or look it up online. Make it a habit to always check if the food is safe to eat or not. If it's not okay to eat, put it in the box, ready to get removed from the house.
4. After collecting all the sugary foods in your box, what you do with them will depend on your circumstances. If the foods belong to other members of your household who are still eating these types of foods, you might need to keep them, in which case I suggest you distinctly mark items as belonging to someone else. The clearer the division is, the more likely you are to resist the temptation.

You may well still be feeling tempted to eat something sugary — just one couldn't hurt, could it?

Remember, focusing on the "why" that you identified on Day One will remind you how important giving up sugar is for you.

But don't beat yourself up if you lose motivation and give in. It's not the end of your journey to being sugar-free, though you may have made it a little harder for yourself. Just get back on the bike and keep going.

Chapter 6

Day Six: Avoiding Sugar Doesn't Mean Avoiding Eating Out

Welcome to Day Six — the second half of your sugar detox challenge!

You're halfway through the challenge, and hopefully, you're feeling significantly better today. If you've been experiencing symptoms that felt like cold or flu, they should be subsiding by now. Soon, you should start feeling the benefits of being sugar-free instead of suffering from withdrawal symptoms.

It might be difficult to stay focused when feeling grotty, but it is important to remember why you are doing it. Your old habits might still be lurking, waiting for your guard to drop; therefore, paying attention to everything you eat and drink is vital until saying no to sugar becomes second nature.

Socialising and having meals out when following a sugar-free diet could be challenging. I know it as I've been there myself. So today, we'll look at how you can stay sugar-free while eating out. I'll give you an overview of which restaurant foods are likely to contain added sugar and explain various strategies to follow so that your dining out experience is smooth.

We'll also be looking at social events, and I'll offer you some suggestions to make sure you're sticking to the sugar-free diet when attending them. Finally, your task today will be to find sugar-free places to eat out. And if you are someone who likes eating out, this will be an extremely useful exercise to do.

Restaurant Foods that Contain Sugar

You probably don't need to be told that some restaurant foods are packed with added sugar. Desserts such as ice cream, crème brûlés or fruit drenched in syrup are perhaps the most obvious. These are just a few types of foods usually loaded with sugar that first come to mind. But plenty of other desserts also have sugar, even if they're not so obviously sweet. For instance, a fruit pie will typically have added sugar in the pastry, and there'll be plenty more if you serve it with cream, ice cream or custard.

The only desserts that won't contain added sugar will be fresh fruit (including fresh fruit salads).

I want to warn you about sugar in fast foods. Your favourite burger, for instance, will have added sugar in the bun, the ketchup and the mayonnaise, at the very least, and that's going to be true of most fast foods, even those that are advertised as "healthy".

What about Chinese, Indian, Italian or other restaurants? The amount of sugar in foods will depend on how it's prepared. But you could assume that the most generic dishes will contain added sugar. Sweet and sour sauce is one of them as well as a korma sauce. Most sauces are usually packed with sugar, so I'd strongly suggest you research the dishes you like eating.

When eating in restaurants, the safest bet is to choose a piece of meat and two veggies or order a salad. But unfortunately, even these foods cannot be guaranteed to be sugar-free. The traditional sauces, such as apple sauce or cranberry sauce, will be made with added sugar too, and if the gravy has been made with granules such as Bisto, it will also contain sugar.

We cannot even trust salads to always be sugar-free. The natural ingredients will be fine, but we don't know what goes into the dressing they put on the salad. It's not only mayonnaise or the salad cream containing sugar — sauces based on oil or vinegar can also have sugary ingredients. For example, if you order a Caesar Salad, you'll get around 3.5g of sugar in a 53g serving of the sauce, and that's almost a teaspoon of sugar.

We're at the end of this section, and you probably feel it's impossible to avoid added sugar when eating out, aren't you? So, what is the solution? Is it to never set foot in a restaurant again? Of course not! That would be rather extreme. I have the solution for you, which I'll discuss in the next section.

How to Avoid Sugar When Eating Out

When I first gave up sugar, I thought I'd be saying goodbye to eating out, which was almost enough to prevent me from going through with it. Health is important, but you need a social life too. I did some research, and fortunately, I discovered in time that there are plenty of ways to enjoy good restaurant foods and stay sugar-free. It just takes a little extra work.

There are two fundamental issues here — how to choose the right restaurant for yourself and how to make sugar-free choices if someone else has picked the restaurant.

Some places you might have already guessed are best avoided, include most, if not all, fast food stores, places where the food is mass-produced in advance and merely cooked on-site (e.g. burgers, fried chicken), and any "production-line" restaurants, where they most likely take all the shortcuts. And shortcuts usually mean added sugar.

On the other hand, just because a restaurant advertises itself as "healthy" doesn't mean it's sugar-free. For instance, you might assume a vegan restaurant is a good candidate. It may be — but bear in mind that most sugar is plant-based and would therefore qualify as vegan.

The same is true of restaurants offering gluten-free, whole-food or low-fat menus. Any of these may well be an excellent place to begin since the owners are thinking about healthy eating, but you'll still need to do your research.

A good start would be simply to google for restaurants in your area and make a list of the results, ignoring any that aren't going to be sugar-free. Then the work begins.

When researching, pay attention to what the website says about the restaurant's aims and methods. If they stress "healthy food" or "traditional cooking", it should be worth checking their menus. Most restaurants will display their menus on their site, so check them out. You already know what to look for and what to avoid from the knowledge you gained from this book. You should be able to judge whether the restaurant food contains sugar or not, whether it's good for you or not.

For example, an Italian restaurant I've just looked up offers a dish containing "Tagliatelle pasta with smoked salmon, served with creamy tomato sauce." Do you remember what I said about sauces? Creamy tomato sauce could potentially hide plenty of added sugar.

Nevertheless, looking at this particular menu, it certainly includes some dishes that look hopeful, so I would have it on the provisional list of "safe to visit" or "sugar-free restaurants", along with any place offering freshly cooked natural ingredients. You could also put Chinese and Indian restaurants on the list, but only if they seem to take health seriously.

Looking at the menu of each restaurant in your local area will give you a clue whether the restaurant is worth visiting or not. A word of advice — your local takeaway is unlikely to be sugar-free.

You could phone the restaurant up and explain that you're hoping to visit but need to avoid added sugar. If possible, speak to the chef since they will be more familiar with the ingredients they use when cooking than the receptionist or the waiter. But, whoever you talk to, try and get them to be specific. A bland "all our food is sugar-free" would be hard to believe, but if they detail half-a-dozen dishes they guarantee to be sugar-free, you're probably on safer ground. And don't forget to question them about items like sauces and gravy.

Eventually, you could build up a database of local restaurants that are safe to visit and mark dishes on their menus that are likely to be sugar-free. You may find many restaurants in your local area that are a part of the big restaurant chains, which will make your job easier when visiting restaurants outside your local area.

Remember, when searching for a restaurant, pick one that seems health-conscious or prides itself on traditional cooking. You may be able to pick out likely foods from the menu based on what you've learnt from this book and your research, but you could also ask the restaurant staff for advice. If you've picked a healthy-eating place, they should be glad to help you choose the meal that suits your needs.

The same advice applies to situations when you don't have a say. This is likely to happen at birthdays, Christmas parties, weddings, or when you are abroad on holiday, where you might struggle to interpret the menus.

Do you have to refuse to go out? Not at all.

What to do in this situation will be discussed in the next section.

Social Events and Avoiding Sugar

When I decided to go sugar-free, I found social events such as parties or receptions even more challenging than going to restaurants. I felt that I had at least some choice when ordering foods from the restaurant menu while having food served to me or laid out as a buffet was out of my control, and I felt that I had no choice in what I was going to eat.

Fortunately, I was given some invaluable advice — never go to a social event hungry.

This does not mean you should eat a lot and then eat nothing at the event, but taking the edge off your hunger with some healthy food beforehand and drinking plenty of water will help you think before you eat.

Whether it is a personal event or something more formal, you can prepare yourself in advance and check the menu before you get there. And if the menu is not available, then perhaps you could contact the organiser in advance and ask about the food options.

Remember, special diets are widely acknowledged nowadays, and hosts may well be getting queries from people needing everything from religious diets to vegan or keto requirements. Making a query about sugar could just be one more.

If it's something you've had to book or formally RSVP, there may even be the option to state any special dietary requirements, and you can clarify that you're on a sugar-free diet.

Whatever the point of contact is, make it clear that you're not necessarily asking for special treatment, just that you need to be able to choose sugar-free options.

Remember, whenever the sugar-free option is available, you need to be aware of how easily sugar can be disguised in foods. Sugar-free food might not be free unless you eat all-natural foods without any sauces or additives.

Besides not arriving hungry at the event, your best approach is to brush up on your lists of safe and unsafe foods, so choosing the right foods for you will become second nature and an easy thing to do even in the whirl of the event.

The advice I share with you in this book should equip you with enough knowledge to enjoy eating out without compromising your sugar-free journey. Just remember, once you've detoxed, as long as it's an occasional occurrence, accept that eating added sugar from time to time and in small quantities is a part of a healthy diet.

Day Six Task: Find Sugar-Free Places for Eating Out Near You

Your sugar withdrawal symptoms are hopefully subsiding. As long as you stay on course, this stage should be nearly over, and you'll start to feel the real benefits of giving up sugar.

To get you there, your task for today will be to find sugar-free places for eating out near you.

Of course, how you define "near you" will depend on where you live and how far you like to travel. For instance, there may be plenty of places within easy walking distance if you're in a city centre, whereas you may need to go further if you live in a village.

There's no right or wrong; choose what suits you best by following these steps:

1. Make a list of restaurants in your local area, however you define that. The easiest way would be a google search, but if you have another way of accessing the options, that's fine.
2. Cross off the unsuitable ones, such as fast-food outlets. You should be able to identify most of these by now.
3. For each possible place, go on their website and read through what they say about themselves. Do they cook fresh food? Do they make a point of healthy eating? These are hopeful signs, though not conclusive.
4. For each place, find the menu on their website. Go through it and identify any meal you think might be sugar-free from what you've learned. If you have difficulty finding any, cross the place off your list.
5. If the dish includes items you're unsure of, look them up online and find out whether they're likely to have hidden sugar, using the information you've learned.

If you prefer, you can phone the restaurants to find out more about any sugar-free dishes they prepare, but this could be left until you're planning a visit.

After the first step, you'll have a much shorter list than when you started. Add notes for each restaurant, including promising meals or the meals you may have doubts about, and keep them somewhere you can easily find them for the next time you want to eat out.

Tomorrow, we'll be moving away from food and focusing on you.

Eating can be motivated by physical hunger as much as triggered by emotions, and we'll examine how emotional eating may affect your sugar-free diet. In the meantime, keep eating healthily and watch out for sugar trying to ambush you.

Chapter 7

Day Seven: The Role of Sugar in Emotional Eating

Welcome to Day Seven of your journey to living sugar-free!

With any luck, the benefits of giving up added sugar will be starting to overhaul the withdrawal symptoms now — the headaches and flu-like symptoms should be clearing up if they haven't already gone. But you might notice that the efforts of your first week could be leaving you exhausted, and you could be feeling tempted to start eating sugar again.

Monday is a new beginning in most people's lives, and many of us tend to make a fresh start on Monday mornings, whether it's a new diet, training regime, weight loss programme, or sugar-free challenge. If you began your 10 Day sugar detox on Monday, this would be your first weekend of being sugar-free.

It's not unusual to see people struggling with sugar-free weekends. And you might find yourself letting your guard down and slipping up today. I know you don't want to do it as you might feel like you're ruining what you've achieved so far, but if it happens, treat it as a learning experience rather than a failure.

Slip-ups are a part of life, but feeling like a failure is a part of self-criticism and shouldn't be encouraged.

Today, instead of looking at the food, the focus is on you. Self-reflection is essential for creating change and making your new habits last.

I often work with people who turn to food whenever they experience any feelings of discomfort. Feeling tired, angry, lonely, bored or anxious are usually the primary triggers of eating unhealthily.

I aim to help you discover what emotional eating is and how your emotions have affected your eating in the past. You'll also learn what common triggers for turning to sugar are, and in today's task, you'll identify your personal sugar triggers.

What is Emotional Eating?

I remember a time (before I began to practice healthy eating, let alone write about it) when I was feeling very down one evening. My "solution" was to go through an entire box of chocolates. Doing that made me feel a lot better for a while. But it didn't last long.

Before long, I was feeling down again. Additionally, I felt guilty for bingeing on all those chocolates — not to mention feeling a bit sick. While this binge eating helped in the short-term, it wasn't a lasting solution for feeling down, sad, and depressed.

Although it may not necessarily have been chocolate, you probably have had similar experiences. Your "comfort food" could be cake or ice cream, pizza or crisps, or any other unhealthy choice that makes you feel better when you eat it, at least for a while.

This type of behaviour is not uncommon. Feeling stressed or upset is often a trigger that leads to an overwhelming urge to eat.

Many clients come to see me because they have developed the habit of overeating their comfort foods due to their emotional state. These foods are almost always unhealthy and, therefore, affect them negatively. Their physical health and emotional well-being suffer, and they often feel like they have lost control over the food they eat.

If you feel like food is controlling you and that certain feelings increase your need to eat comfort foods (interestingly, people rarely turn to broccoli or salad when feeling stressed or upset), I can reassure you that this isn't just "all in your mind".

Food can affect your brain chemistry and alter your moods. And when you're feeling anxious or upset, your brain interprets this as a threat and prepares for fight or flight, the same as when a sabre-tooth tiger threatened our distant ancestors.

The fight or flight response includes stocking up on energy-producing foods — and, as you now are aware, sugar's primary role in its natural state is to provide energy for the brain and muscles. However, as you have nothing to fight or flee from in the modern world, and the diet that we live on is often packed with foods containing added sugar, the energy isn't used up. The free sugar in what you've eaten creates the cycle of a sugar rush, followed by low moods and more cravings for sugary foods.

So how do you recognise whether you're an emotional eater? Here are several signs:

- Eating more when you feel stressed
- Eating when you're not hungry
- Eating to make yourself feel better
- Using food to reward yourself
- Eating till you feel bloated
- Feeling safe with food
- Being out of control with food

Any of these can be a sign you're an emotional eater — and, as the type of foods you turn to are likely to be sugary, failing to deal with emotional eating can quickly get you off track when following your sugar-free programme.

Sugar and Dopamine

As you know, sugar is an addictive substance; it's been shown to be more addictive than cocaine. This is mainly due to a chemical process in the brain that produces dopamine.

Dopamine is often characterised as the brain's "pleasure and reward" chemical. This is an oversimplification, but its role in addiction is essentially just that. The brain releases dopamine when it recognises behaviour that needs to be encouraged, producing a high level of joy. For example, the brain recognises sex as positive for the species' survival and ensures that the organism associates sex with pleasure.

This is a positive thing, although it's not beneficial to us when we crave an experience in the wrong context. But addictive drugs such as heroin and cocaine will use this process against us by artificially stimulating dopamine production, leading us to crave more of the substance.

Several studies have shown that sugar has the same effect.[15] [16] This is because it's a high-calorie food to provide us with energy. Over perhaps a thousand generations, human brains have learned to reward eating sugar with a dopamine rush, which in turn, increased sugar cravings. We benefited from it for most of human history since our ancestors needed the high energy reserves as they never knew when they'd next have access to such food.

In modern times, unfortunately, this is no longer appropriate. It can lead to sugar addiction.

The brain "knows" the very thing that will cheer us up — the dopamine rush from indulging in sugary foods. And in a world where sugar is everywhere, and the foods we consume are primarily processed instead of eaten in the natural form, we are now witnessing adverse effects on our health.

As you're reading this book, you're probably better informed about your sugar cravings or addiction than most people out there, but recognising your triggers might still be an issue for you.

In the next section, we will look at the most commonly experienced triggers, and then in the chapter task, you'll be encouraged to look at what triggers you to eat sugar.

Common Sugar Triggers

Have you ever walked by a vending machine and seen a chocolate bar? So you took a few coins from your purse and bought your favourite type?

Or what about having a stressful day at work, and on the way home, you needed something sweet to cheer you up?

There are various types of sugar triggers.

Each individual has different triggers depending mainly on the kind of life they lead and what situations they're susceptible to.

Passing the vending machine could be a significant sugar trigger for some people or being surrounded by all the sweet stuff at the checkout in the supermarket. On the other hand, feeling tired, stressed or anxious could also lead to eating sugar. As discussed previously, some people have difficulty dealing with emotional upsets, and seeking comfort in food is not uncommon.

Anything that causes stress or upset can be a sugar trigger, such as feeling bored, lonely, anxious or overwhelmed. They can all be a cause for eating sugar. There's no right or wrong answer.

To some people, preparing for an exam or an important meeting can be seen as a traumatic event and enough to trigger the need to eat sugar. While to others, it might be just a minor annoyance that doesn't cause any damaging effect.

On the other hand, a trigger can also be something that seems positive.

Some people use sugar as a reward for an achievement or associate it with relaxation after a busy period. If this is very occasional and well-defined (e.g. Christmas), it may not be too severe and cause any significant issues, but the danger is that your brain, wanting the reward, will start identifying more and more occasions as being "like Christmas".

Some of the most common types of sugar triggers include:

- *Stress*: The production of cortisol in the brain caused by stress makes you seek out high-energy food such as sugar and the dopamine reward to counteract your bad mood.
- *Negative emotions*: Eating can be a way to temporarily take your mind off negative emotions such as anxiety, loneliness, fear, shame or anger.
- *Boredom*: If you're feeling bored, eating will occupy your attention for a while, distracting you from the more fundamental issues that may have created the boredom.
- *Childhood conditioning*: Did your well-meaning parents use food to reward you? If so, you can be sure it was high-sugar food, and you've become conditioned to see that kind of food as a way to feel positive.
- *Social influences*: If all your most enjoyable social situations are connected with eating unhealthy food like pizza or chips with several spoons of tomato ketchup, the enjoyment of being with your friends can transfer to the food itself.

Day Seven Task: Identify Your Sugar Triggers

Your first Seven Days of the sugar-free programme are over.

How are you feeling?

If everything goes as planned, you should feel much more positive than a few days ago. And if you've had a slip-up, don't worry too much — just get yourself back to sugar-free eating.

Today, we looked at the common sugar triggers, and in this task, your job will be to identify your triggers. Your sugar triggers might be much more specific to you and your circumstances. Perhaps, you are constantly bingeing on sugar on Friday evening after having a stressful week at work, or on a particular day out with a group of friends, or perhaps when the afternoon at work seems endless.

Your task today is to go to the Workbook and follow these steps:

1. Take some time to think about all the times you can remember over the past few weeks when you've mainly indulged in food or drink you now recognise as sugary, and describe each occasion. There is a space provided in the Workbook to write your answers.
2. Go through your list and group the occasions into similar situations, giving each a simple name (e.g. "Friday Night Flop", "Quiz Night", "Sunday Brunch", "Sleepless Night", "Stressful Event", etc.).
3. Write down a few notes about each of these situations to identify what it was about them that led you to eat sugar. It was probably broadly connected with one of the triggers I have already mentioned in the previous

section of this book, but it was unique to you.

Whatever answers you wrote down are likely to be your primary sugar triggers. Although, bear in mind that something which hasn't happened for some time could be a risk too.

Your trigger list should be a tool to help you think more clearly about what triggers you to eat sugary foods so you can plan how to avoid falling into the trap.

Identifying your triggers and combining them with mindful eating could be a powerful tool in gaining control over your unconscious bad habits — and bad eating habits are no exception. That is what we'll be looking at tomorrow. I'll explain the importance of mindful eating and how it can help you avoid sugar in your diet.

Chapter 8

Day Eight: Mindful Eating

Welcome to Day Eight of your programme to go sugar-free!

After all the improvements over the past couple of days, you may be getting some discouragement from your body today. Most typically, this is likely to come in the form of digestive problems — either constipation or diarrhoea, depending on how your body will react to the changes it's going through. But don't panic — it's your digestive system clearing out the toxins associated with high sugar consumption so it can start functioning properly. While it can be very uncomfortable for a day or two, it's actually your gut adjusting to your new diet.

The problem is likely to be an increase in insoluble fibre from the vegetables you've started to add to your diet.

If this is leading to constipation, you can:

- Eat vegetables like carrots, parsnips or sweet potatoes at least twice a day
- Eat vegetables containing prebiotic fibre (e.g. asparagus, onion, garlic)
- Eat starches (e.g. legumes, brown rice, white potatoes) that have been boiled and then left to cool

If your problem is diarrhoea, you can:

- Drink peppermint, camomile or ginger tea
- Eat more fermented food (e.g. pickles)
- Eat fennel, either raw or cooked
- Avoid leafy greens, nuts, seeds and legumes
- Take an L-glutamine supplement and a high-quality probiotic (seek advice from your doctor before taking any supplements. This particularly applies to you if you're on any medication)

Today, we'll look at mindful eating, its benefits, and how it can help you avoid sugar. At the end of the chapter, you'll be practising mindful eating, which will give you a practical demonstration of how it can help you.

What is Mindful Eating?

Mindful eating is an in-the-moment awareness of the food and drinks you consume. It is a technique that allows you to focus attention only on the present, tuning out all the thoughts that might distract you. It derives mainly from Buddhist meditation practices, but you can practice mindfulness without any spiritual aspect.

People who have heard of mindful eating but don't know much about it often think it's all about chewing food slowly. While that's a valuable technique used in mindful eating, it is not the main focus.

Think about your mealtimes. What are they like? Do you most often eat alone or together with family or friends? If you have traditional family dinners, the chances are that you're chatting the whole time. It's the same if you go to lunch with your work colleagues. It's understandable, of course. Mealtimes have always been the perfect opportunity for people to deepen relationships with one another — but these situations don't leave much chance to concentrate on the food you're putting in your body.

Often, people eat while they are watching TV. It's an excellent chance to multi-tasking, but how often have you finished watching a TV programme, found an empty plate in front of you, and had no memory of what the meal tasted like?

On the other hand, do you mix mealtimes with work? This can be a particular problem at lunchtime or when snacking. "There's so much to do", you say. "Maybe it's best just to bring the food to the desk and carry on working?" and that's what you do. Even if you leave your desk, it's difficult to escape from the phone, isn't it? So half your lunch break consists of taking calls.

And yes, I've experienced all of these. It's very easy to fall into the trap of eating mindlessly when not eating mindfully. And it's tough to practise mindful eating during social occasions. When conversing with another person, we tend to focus on what we are saying or hearing rather than what we are doing.

When eating mindlessly, I often overeat or eat food that does not benefit my body. On the other hand, when eating mindfully, it extends well beyond the actual process of eating. This means that:

- I use my inner wisdom in selecting and preparing food to nurture myself
- I use all my senses to choose food that will both

nourish me and that I'll enjoy
- I respond to whether I like or dislike food (or neither) without pre-judgement
- I am aware of hunger and satiety cues, allowing me to know when to eat and when to stop

The good news is that none of this rules out sharing a meal with family or friends. It helps, of course, if the people you're eating with are aware that you're practising mindful eating, so when they ask you questions during the meal, you are not expected to respond immediately.

However, to eat mindfully, it is best to avoid other distractions. When you have a break at work for lunch or snacks, leave your desk — and put that phone on silent. For meals at home, keep the TV or games console off. Multi-tasking may be considered a good thing, but that doesn't apply when learning to live mindfully.

Benefits of Mindful Eating

Why eat mindfully?

So far, some of what I've said should have given significant clues as to why eating mindfully is a good thing. Awareness of when you need to eat and when you're full is crucial for sticking to a healthy diet, especially if you're vulnerable to emotional eating or bingeing. The best way to eat healthily is to eat enough, but not too much, and eat regularly — mindful eating is a vital tool to help you do this.

Your body is a beautiful thing that can tell you precisely what you need to eat. The trouble is, this process can often go wrong (especially when living in a world very different from the one we were designed for). Your instincts can sometimes tell you to eat food that's bad for you.

You've already seen how this can happen with sugar. For instance, your brain still thinks you must fight or flee from a dangerous animal when you get stressed, preparing you for it. The instincts you should be able to rely on are often geared to what you would have needed twenty thousand years ago, rather than today.

Suppose you pay attention to what you're eating, staying in the present instead of letting your mind wander. In this case, you can learn to ignore the false cues and focus on the true ones — including, crucially, recognising when you've eaten enough.

In the same way, a mindful choice of food can help you select items that are good for you and provide your body with what it needs. Conscious decisions can range from the type of food selected (e.g. fruit rather than sweets) to choosing a healthy portion size.

This process may have to cut through your preconceptions. You might have decided as a child that you don't like broccoli, for instance. This might be because your parents didn't like it, so you assumed it was horrible.

Being non-judgemental about the food you try can help break through these assumptions. So, you might try spinach mindfully and still decide you don't like it. That's all right — you can find an alternative with similar benefits. On the other hand, you might be surprised to find that something you always thought you hated is quite pleasant.

Mindful eating has been successfully used to help people escape from emotional eating and binge eating, but even if these aren't problems for you, it can still help in other ways, such as aiding digestion. Studies have also found an apparent connection between mindful eating and successful weight loss, although more research is needed to confirm this.[17]

More generally, mindful eating has been associated with increased psychological well-being, reduced risk of chronic diseases (through better food choices and digestion) — and not to mention greater enjoyment of the food you eat.

How can Mindful Eating Help with Sugar Consumption?

The biggest problem with sugar is that it's so easy to eat without thinking about it. It can be found in many food items and drinks, even when they're not obviously sweet. And when you are not paying attention, it is easy to reach for something with sugar.

This is far more of a problem than it would have been one hundred years ago. Not only are most of us in a rush all the time today, with no time to think about what we're choosing, but the food is far easier to pick up without thought. We no longer have to go through the process of buying the food, preparing and cooking it, which would give us time to think about what's in it. Instead, we can just pop into the nearest shop or put a coin in a vending machine, giving us instant gratification.

Of course, someone who isn't aware of the problems that sugar can cause or simply doesn't care won't be bothered by any of this. This problem can come up if you're trying to give up sugar — being unmindful about your eating can result in eating something sugary simply because you're too distracted to think about it.

Mindful eating encourages you to be always conscious of what you're eating, from the first recognition that you're hungry right through to swallowing — and beyond. As far as your choice of food or drink is concerned, your mindfulness practice will, eventually, make it second nature to stop and think about what you're considering, whether it's good for you, and what choice will be both nutritious and enjoyable.

It will also make you think about whether you are really hungry. We're all creatures of habit, and a lot of the time, these habits help us navigate our busy schedules — as long as they're the right ones. The problem comes when we've developed bad habits (or at least unnecessary ones) and keep doing them because it's easier than challenging them.

Mindfulness can help us challenge negative habits in many areas of our lives, and applying mindfulness practices around eating and drinking can certainly benefit us. If you've always gone to the vending machine or the nearest shop around 4 p.m. to get a coke and a chocolate bar, the first thing to be aware of is whether you're doing it because you're hungry or if it's a learned behaviour.

It's essential to take time and get in touch with what your body is telling you. If your mindful self concludes that you are hungry, you can choose how to respond to it instead of reacting to it on autopilot. When you stop and get in touch with your body's needs, your mindful state will allow you to consider what would make a good, healthy alternative that you'll enjoy just as much — if not more.

If you conclude that you aren't hungry at all but are mindlessly snacking due to the response to an old habit, you could develop an alternative healthy habit that will bring more benefits to your life.

As I've already discussed, many foods disguise their sugar effectively, and a mindless approach to choice and preparation can allow something sugary to slip through your attention. Being mindful about choosing and preparing your ingredients will enable you to review what you know about the item and decide whether it's something you want to have in your diet.

The benefits of mindful eating to your sugar-free diet aren't restricted to choosing what to eat and when. Although your body's uptake of natural sugars, such as those in fresh fruit and vegetables, should be healthy, wolfing the food down while your mind is elsewhere could make this less effective.

Mindful eating encourages you to eat slowly and deliberately, savouring each mouthful. This will help make your digestion more effective, including how your body processes the natural sugars in food.

The other reason mindful eating is beneficial is that it provides a great range of healthy options for your sugar-free diet. As I mentioned earlier, most of us make assumptions about not liking certain foods, often things we've never really given a chance — and, more often than not, these are the healthy foods we need to eat.

Mindful eating allows you to assess these items realistically. When you're focusing entirely on the present, there's no room to think about your past assumptions or anticipate how you might dislike the taste. It gives you the freedom to decide what you really think about it.

That doesn't mean, of course, that you'll love every food you try. We all have individual tastes, and perhaps you had a good reason to avoid certain foods. However, you might be surprised to find out how many foods you've "always hated" that aren't so bad. Perhaps some may even turn into new favourites.

And this will be necessary. With so many old favourites that you now realise contain alarming amounts of free sugar, you'll need new favourites to take their place — and you may well find them among foods you've always avoided.

Day Eight Task: Practice Mindful Eating

Today, it's all about mindful eating. Your task is to plan, prepare and eat your meal on your own and without any external distractions. Once mindful eating is part of your regular practice, this won't be necessary, but while you're learning to develop your new habit, it's important to know how to cut yourself off from the outside world.

Your task includes setting time aside to plan your meal. And if you meditate, it would be helpful to do so at the start of the session to get you focused.

Focus entirely on yourself in the present moment, not allowing thoughts of the past or the future to break in. Then move your thinking to the food and start planning in your mind what you want to eat, eliminating all sugary foods.

By now, you should know which foods are sugar-free and belong to the safe group and which ones contain sugar and hence belong to the unsafe group. If in doubt, go to the Workbook, and check your answers on Day Two.

When ready, go into the kitchen on your own and without distractions. Maybe you have a kitchen routine — listening to the radio or putting the TV on. These habits might not distract you once you're used to mindfulness, but right now you want to be able to focus entirely on each task at hand during food preparation. Removing any external distractions and staying in the present is necessary while chopping vegetables, cooking, and smelling the aroma of the food. This is a great way to practise mindfulness and stay in the present. We often live in the past or think about the future. Focusing on the present moment is a powerful place to be.

When you start eating, take your time. Chew each mouthful slowly, savouring the taste and texture of the food. Think about what it tastes like and what you think of it, without reaching back into your memory to identify your preconceptions about what you're eating. If one particular ingredient from the food doesn't appeal to you, think about the taste and find the words to describe it.

After the meal, take some time to reflect on the experience and note your reactions:

- Was there anything you enjoyed better than before — especially anything you've consciously avoided?
- Or was there anything you didn't particularly like about the meal — a texture, smell, taste, etc.?
- Have you noticed anything unusual? (If you did, it might be because you've always eaten it without real thought). What have you noticed?

Of course, you won't have to go through this process for every meal for the rest of your life. Eventually, you'll be able to slip into mindful eating whenever you need to and process the information you receive quickly, but for this exercise, take your time.

Over the next few days, I encourage you to allocate one meal a day when you will consciously choose to eat mindfully and follow the process outlined in today's task.

Chapter 9

Day Nine: Dealing with Sugar Cravings

Welcome to Day Nine of your Sugar Detox Challenge!

If you were suffering from digestion issues yesterday and took my advice about the foods to target, hopefully, your digestion has improved. And if your first attempt at mindful eating was unsuccessful, don't worry — with practice, you will become an expert. As you get used to cooking with natural ingredients instead of just heating up ready-made meals or relying on sugary snacks to keep you going through the day, the knowledge you gained and the mindfulness lesson from yesterday will make this process much easier and more enjoyable.

Whether your goal to quit sugar is to improve your health, lose weight, or both, you'll notice positive changes. But one of the biggest problems going sugar-free that people often face is — sugar cravings. You've got through the first week of your detox on your initial enthusiasm, but that may be wearing a little thin by now, and you may be experiencing a strong desire to go back to eating sugar.

This will be the topic of today's lesson.

I'll explain sugar cravings and what happens to your body when you experience them. You'll learn to overpower and avoid bad habits and situations where you're likely to lose focus. I'll also recommend some sugarless desserts that you can make, and finally, you'll be putting your learning into practice.

What are Sugar Cravings?

Sugar cravings aren't just wanting sugar because you enjoy it. Yes, there are times when we all experience that. Let's face it, for generations, even our ancestors were taught that sweet things taste good, and sometimes we might fancy the taste of something sweet. But cravings are far more than that. It is when you desperately need to eat something sugary — or, more likely, you need some particular sugary food. This is because your brain translates a general need for sugar into a specific need for something effective in fulfilling that need in the past.

Our brains remember things and feelings, which create a need for a sugar rush and the dopamine reward. And when sugar cravings kick in, it's very tempting to give in. That's why learning strategies to deal with cravings is essential so that you can manage them better.

Years ago, I was addicted to sugar, and my cravings were very powerful. I tried various things, and learning about them helped me understand what was happening in my body when I experienced an overwhelming need for sugar.

If you are in a situation where you feel like you'll never get over it and you'll always be at the mercy of your sugar cravings, believe me, eliminating added sugar from your diet will get you on the right track. Your body will adapt to the more proportionate dopamine levels from the natural sugars, and you will say goodbye to the crashes that follow the highs and the cravings that go with them. And that's what you have to look forward to if you stick to your sugar-free detox for two more days.

What Happens in the Body When You Have Cravings?

There are various reasons why we experience sugar cravings. Sugar is addictive, and the desire to have sugar is no different from other addictions.

I remember when I felt such intense cravings for sugary foods that there was nothing that could stop me from wanting it. Sugar was all I could think of.

I was at a work meeting once that lasted for hours. After a couple of hours of being stuck in the room with my colleagues, smokers started fidgeting, and I was the same. We could not wait for the meeting to finish so that we could all go outside. The smokers went for a cigarette, and I went to the local shop to buy a chocolate bar. Once I felt the taste of chocolate melting inside my mouth, I felt fine. I was happy. I felt myself again.

When we feed our bodies with natural sugar from fresh fruit or vegetables, the glucose gets channelled to the muscles and brain as a steady, moderate flow and is converted into the energy we need. This generates the feel-good hormone dopamine in small quantities, providing the brain with just enough satisfaction.

On the other hand, free sugars found in most packaged foods, particularly in sweets, cakes and chocolates, cause a massive rush of glucose to the brain, producing far more energy than we can use and causing the "sugar rush" familiar in children who consume too many sweets or fizzy drinks. This creates a massive rush of dopamine which means that the brain associates eating sugary food with pleasure and desperately wants it again. There's evidence that the effects of free sugar can change the brain's chemistry, making regular intake essential for its functioning.[18]

This is especially dangerous when we feel stressed, as that's when — apart from a heightened need for that dopamine rush — the body is also preparing for a fight or flight response, directing us to stock up on energy. And as you've learned, the most immediate energy source is sugar.

Another factor in sugar cravings is that free sugar can interfere with the normal functioning of the appetite hormones called ghrelin. Ghrelin gives the signal to the brain indicating hunger. On the other hand, leptin, another hormone associated with food and eating, tells you when you've had enough.

The effects of sugar addiction can be that ghrelin is being produced, even when we don't need to eat, and the resulting illusion of hunger can combine with signals from the brain, which lead to intense sugar cravings.

Ways to Overcome Sugar Cravings

After deciding to give up sugar, I desperately wanted the foods I was trying to avoid.

I remember experiencing intense cravings and struggling to overcome a strong desire to taste something sweet in my mouth.

I now know that sugar cravings are one of the withdrawal symptoms that we feel when we want to quit eating sugar.

At the time, I had just started to do my training in nutrition, and I was aware of some very effective strategies for overcoming cravings which I began to apply.

The simplest way to beat sugar cravings is to eat healthily and follow a balanced diet of various food types. Healthy sources include fibre-rich foods and healthy fats. The presence of fibre and healthy fats with natural sugar helps the body process natural sugars steadily. This will prevent you from experiencing a sugar rush followed by a sudden crash, which is very common when eating a large amount of processed food and following a western diet. A lousy diet often leaves you wanting more foods and needing more sugar.

One of the tips that my clients benefit from is regular eating. This means having a meal or snack every three to four hours. I'm aware of the advice recommending the opposite and not having meals too close to one another, but balancing the blood sugar levels through regular eating and consuming healthy foods will prevent you from being too hungry. It will also discourage you from turning to sugary snacks when feeling peckish or experiencing low energy levels. Also, as I have already mentioned, regular eating, including fibre, healthy fats and protein, is an integral part of a healthy diet that can help you regulate your glucose level and stop you from wanting more foods loaded with sugar and simple carbs.

I always suggest to my clients to get familiar with their snacking behaviours. If your routine involves eating something you're craving, then changing your habits and practices can help avoid the temptation.

You learned yesterday about the effectiveness of mindfulness and the ways it can help you eat healthily. Fighting cravings is no exception. When you experience cravings, I suggest you try meditating or breathing exercises. It will bring you back into the present, where you can consciously decide whether a piece of chocolate or a pack of five doughnuts is something you need at that moment.

Doing something you like can help you fight your sugar-craving habits. Some of the things you may want to try could be listening to your favourite music or going for a brisk walk. Whatever you choose to do, focus all your attention on it and make it a habit. Replacing unhealthy behaviours with healthy ones can make a big difference if you apply them every time you experience cravings.

Using the strategy of doing something you like and helping you feel rewarded will reduce your sugar cravings and raise your dopamine level. It will boost your dopamine naturally and make your brain less interested in getting its fix from sugar.

Bad Habits Related to Sugar

If I were to ask you, "What habits do you have that lead you to overeat sugar?" what would be your response?

Before reading this book, you might have struggled to get anything further than "sometimes I eat chocolates".

I believe that by now, you are aware that there's more to sugar consumption than simply eating a bar of chocolate once in a while.

What you eat is as important as how and why you eat.

Here are some of the most damaging behavioural patterns associated with eating sugar:

- *Skipping meals — especially breakfast*: One of the most crucial aspects of regulating a healthy uptake of natural sugar is eating regularly and healthily. Breakfast is vital to set you up for the day, and skipping it will leave your brain demanding the sugar it needs for your energy. The problem is that this is likely to be translated as a craving for something that will deliver a quick sugar rush — chocolate, biscuits, Coke etc. The same is expected to happen if you work through lunchtime and skip it.
- *Mindless snacking*: Life is busy, and reaching for convenient foods when you feel peckish might have become your daily routine. Snacking is essential to a healthy diet, but make sure you apply healthy choices. Making unhealthy choices will not take you to your sugar-free life. Your focus must be on making the right choices, which require your full attention at the start of this journey. Practising mindfulness could turn your

mindless snacking into a mindful force that will give you a stepping stone to a healthier life.

- *Snacking at the same time every day:* Eating at the same time every day isn't uncommon. There's nothing wrong with following the same eating patterns daily if that includes eating healthy foods, but if you keep snacking on sugary products (and this is the issue for many people), then your behaviour will not match your intentions of leading a sugar-free life.
- *Not getting enough sleep*: Yes, this comes up a lot, but the reality is that getting a whole night's sleep regularly is crucial to every aspect of your health. Regular snacking on sugary foods throughout the day can disrupt your hormones and affect your sleep. Skimping on your sleep can disrupt your natural cycles — and that includes your glucose and hunger cycles, which can lead to sugar cravings.
- *Shopping without a list*: This is another one that applies to all healthy eating, and I discussed it on Day Four. You're much more likely to pick up sugary foods if you start buying food on impulse instead of carefully planning it. To avoid this, decide what you'll buy before walking into the shop, and stick to your decision. Preferably, you'll make the grocery list before leaving the house, so you are well-prepared. Also, check nutrition labels if you doubt the sugar content in any product while shopping.

In this section, we discussed the most common habits that can lead to eating sugar. The following section will look at the situations where you are most likely to get disrupted and forget about healthy eating.

Situations Where You're Likely to Lose Focus

There isn't a good time to lower your guard when you're giving up sugar. Until you're thoroughly detoxed, your body can be your enemy, telling you that you need food that will produce the dopamine rush your brain is craving. Before choosing sugar-free foods by preference becomes second nature, you must be careful around food.

There are situations when you can be especially at risk because you have other things on your mind that seem more important than your diet.

For example, social events such as parties or weddings can be challenging. As I've already mentioned, one of the problems with these events is that you're not in control of the menu, and it can be challenging to know whether the food on offer is safe. I've suggested ways to prepare for this, but you might get distracted and not be thinking about it while celebrating.

Similarly, it's easy to lose focus when socialising with friends — especially after a drink or two. Perhaps the best strategy in this situation would be to talk to as many friends as possible about your intentions and express how important it is to you. This makes it more likely that you'll be surrounded by people in such a situation who will be looking out for you.

Apart from being out with your friends and having a good time, you can also risk turning to sugar when busy. That's partly because you don't have the time and attention to think about what you are eating. This is another reason why learning mindfulness can be a powerful tool to help you manage your need for sugary foods.

Being in stressful situations is another major problem for many people. Feeling stressed is one of the most common reasons people grab a chocolate bar on the way home from work or when making plans to do something and expect to get stressed. The need for having sugar when stressed could be because the brain is likely to flashback to its primaeval assumption that stress means to fight or flight — and it is going to need sugar for the energy. But, guess what? Once you master the practice of mindfulness, you'll find yourself paying attention to what you're eating, even when you are feeling overwhelmed with work and other commitments.

Mindfulness exercises could be a great way to manage your eating patterns better, identify what makes you stressed, and understand how you react to your body's prompts.

Day Nine Task: Beat Your Sugar Cravings

How have you been coping with your sugar cravings?

Hopefully, the tips I've given you today have helped you. And if you've given in to something, learn from the experience and develop strategies for successfully resisting temptation in the future.

In today's task, you are going to focus on your sugar cravings by following four simple steps:

1. Remember as many occasions as you can when you have felt cravings since starting your sugar-free

journey nine days ago. Write down in your Workbook when it was, what you were doing, and what you were craving. Don't be worried if you have a long list. That's perfectly normal; the more information you have, the better.

2. Think about each of these occasions and identify whether you were doing something at the time that you generally associate with the food you were craving. If you can't think of anything, that's okay, but be honest with yourself.

3. From what you've learned over the past nine days, identify a list of sugar-free foods that you could substitute for your cravings. Think of something that you like eating or you'd like to try. Make sure you add your ideas to this list whenever you think of sugar-free substitutes.

4. In situations where cravings were connected with a specific problem, identify what you could have done to raise your dopamine levels healthily. Perhaps you could take some time-out and go for a walk, meditate, or read a few pages of your favourite book — pick something that will be a positive experience.

5. In the Workbook, you will find the table that will help you to make a list containing all this information in the format that's easy to follow. The information that you enter in the table will be helpful to you in the future. You can quickly refer to it whenever you start feeling sugar cravings. That will make a big difference to your success.

You're almost at the end of the 10 Day Sugar Detox Challenge — one more day to go, but that won't be the end of your sugar-free journey. Tomorrow, you'll discover what life without sugar can be like and the benefits you'll soon begin to recognise.

In the meantime, good luck with resisting those cravings.

Chapter 10

Day Ten: Life Without Sugar

Congratulations — you've made it to the last day of the Sugar Detox Challenge!

These first ten days were the most crucial to your sugar-free journey. You were introduced to sugar detox, learned about the various places where sugar is hiding, implemented new behaviours that hopefully helped you stay sugar-free, and managed the discomfort of withdrawal symptoms.

It is important to remember that these ten days were just the beginning of your sugar-free life. The challenge will remain until your behaviour becomes automatic and choosing sugar-free foods becomes second nature. But don't get discouraged; it will get much easier from now.

Today, you will be reminded of the health benefits you have to look forward to if you continue with your sugar-free diet. Reminding yourself of all the benefits of living a sugar-free life is your best motivation.

Today, on the final day of the challenge, you'll be looking at how to create various strategies for adopting a sugar-free diet as a permanent part of your life. You'll receive plenty of ideas and helpful advice on planning your meals effectively so that, in time, you won't miss sugar. Another critical point that we'll discuss today will be how committing yourself to carry on with your new lifestyle can play a significant role in successfully continuing your sugar-free diet.

Long-Term Health Benefits of Cutting Down on Sugar

I've talked a lot about the damaging effects of sugar on your body and brain, but what does giving it up mean in the long term?

The longer you continue to live without eating sugar, the more you'll experience health benefits. Here are a few of them:

- *Improved dental health*: Perhaps the most prominent health benefit is improving your dental health. Added sugar is the most significant factor in tooth decay, and while giving it up won't repair existing damage, it will certainly slow down any further deterioration.
- *A healthier heart*: This shouldn't be much of a surprise by now. In 2014, a study suggested that getting 21% of your calories from added sugar found in sugar-sweetened beverages, fruit drinks, dairy desserts, etc. may mean a 38% higher risk of dying from heart disease than if you kept the level of added sugar in your diet to 8%. This appears to be connected with higher blood pressure and bad cholesterol.[19]
- *Losing weight and abdominal fat*: As I've already explained, added sugar affects how insulin regulates glucose in your blood sugar, resulting in extra fat, especially abdominal fat. A long-term healthy diet without added sugar should see the fat falling off.

- *Lower diabetes risk*: Again, this shouldn't be a surprise. The same better-regulated insulin that helps you lose fat will also reduce your risk of developing type 2 diabetes.
- *Good for your brain*: Excessive glucose sent to the brain can affect its functioning and even alter its structure. Studies have suggested that the high consumption of added sugar reduces the effectiveness of brain functions. At the same time, it also inhibits the production of brain-derived neurotrophic factors (BDNF), which is vital for memory. Low levels of BDNF have been associated with the development of Alzheimer's Disease and other types of dementias, so a sugar-free diet may reduce your risk level.[20]
- *Decrease inflammation*: Overeating sugar can lower your immunity and increase inflammation in the body, causing aches and pains in the joints. Quitting sugar can decrease inflammation and support your immune system, helping you feel better.
- *Younger-looking skin*: This is perhaps the most unexpected health benefit of giving up sugar, but there are good reasons. High blood sugar levels inhibit the collagen repair that keeps your skin healthy. Giving up the added sugar can reduce sagging and premature wrinkles, giving you smoother and younger-looking skin.

These are great long-term health benefits that you'll experience if you reduce eating sugar or remove it from your diet altogether. In the next section, you'll learn more tips on how to continue with your new healthy eating habits.

Tips to Continue Eating Less Sugar

Over the last ten days, you've learned what foods and drinks you need to avoid to continue living a sugar-free life. But until it becomes second nature to shop and prepare sugar-free meals and snacks, you may easily slip back into your bad old habits.

Several strategies that you've learned since the beginning of the challenge worth repeating include:

- Continue to practise mindful eating. You learned about this on Day Eight. I'd like you to remember that this is an approach to life, not just during this challenge. If you make everything mindful around the food, such as planning, preparation, and mealtimes, remembering the benefits of remaining sugar-free will be much easier, and you will feel encouraged to continue your new lifestyle.
- Plan your shopping trip so you're not tempted to buy something unsuitable on impulse. Make a list, researching any item you're unsure about — though this will become rarer the longer you've been doing it.
- Make a weekly meal plan, ensuring that everything you include is sugar-free, and even more importantly, give yourself a varied, exciting range of meals that you'll be looking forward to. Bland meals will likely make you miss the sugary food and return to your old habits.
- Concentrate on eating healthily since healthy food is likely without added sugar. Use fresh ingredients as much as possible, and remember to eat the rainbow of fruit and vegetables to get all the necessary vitamins and minerals.

- Get to know the local restaurants that are likely to offer sugar-free or at least low-sugar options, and explore what to choose from the menu if you decide to visit them. This will help you continue living sugar-free without giving up eating out.
- Make sure your family and friends know about and understand what you're doing so that they can back you up instead of putting temptation in your way.
- If you miss something sweet beyond mere cravings, schedule yourself occasional treats. For instance, if you love cakes, allow yourself a small amount on special occasions such as Easter, Christmas, or birthdays.

Moving Beyond the 10 Day Sugar Detox Challenge

Doing the 10 Day Sugar Detox Challenge and keeping the sugar out of your diet has been hard, and you may feel anxious about keeping up that level of effort indefinitely.

I can reassure you that sugar addiction doesn't last forever once you've removed added sugar from your diet and replaced it with the necessary nutrients your body needs. Yes, you may still have a nostalgic feeling of missing the taste, but the intense sugar craving should be gone, and hopefully, you can notice the benefits and feel it has been worth it.

When we stop adding processed sugar to the foods, the brain relearns what it needs, and the lows we used to experience when the sugar rush has run out will no longer be there. Instead, the brain will get used to a steady flow of the glucose needed for healthy functioning and accept natural sources such as sugar from whole fruit, vegetables and dairy as something you should be eating. Removing processed sugar from the diet changes the taste buds, and the body no longer craves it.

If you still experience intense cravings on Day Ten, they may be caused by your mental or emotional state rather than your physical state. As you've learned over the past ten days, bingeing on sugar is often enhanced, if not created, during stress, anxiety or depression, or when experiencing any other negative feelings you struggle to manage.

Doing the sugar detox probably helped you learn things about yourself that you weren't aware of before, including why your body needs sugar or reasons for craving sugary foods when feeling emotional or stressed. Bringing awareness and understanding of your emotional struggles should help you reduce your temptations to emotional eating a bit better.

Nevertheless, this doesn't mean there will be no more work to do when learning about yourself. Inner work is essential to creating or maintaining change in life.

As I've already said before, it's essential to identify what gives you pleasure. When joy is missing, people often search for alternative ways to get dopamine.

Most of my clients find sugar to be a great way to boost their dopamine levels until they realise the foods they eat cannot fill the hole inside them. After spending some time working together and discovering patterns of their unhealthy behaviours, the connection between limiting beliefs and self-sabotage often comes to light.

I often see people struggling to believe in their ability to succeed, and clinging to old beliefs and behaviours makes them safe. Some make significant changes to their lifestyle and adopt healthy routines, but they struggle to maintain their progress. They keep returning to their old self even when holding on to the old patterns is causing them harm.

Do you recognise yourself in this? Letting go of the old beliefs that don't serve you anymore is crucial when changing any area of your life, including removing added sugar from your diet. Giving yourself a label that you're a sugar addict and holding on to it will sabotage your good efforts.

Labelling yourself will permit you to behave in a way that matches your identity label. If you call yourself a sugar addict or someone who loves eating sugary foods, you will struggle to act like someone who is not that person.

To break the behavioural pattern, you must decide who you want to be and start acting like that person. If you wish to continue with the healthy lifestyle and the success you accomplished over the last ten days, you must bring a new identity to support your new lifestyle. This might not align with your old self-beliefs, so it's essential to understand which behaviour — the old or a new one, will bring you closer to or take you further away from your goal.

It isn't enough just to make a behavioural change. No behaviour will last unless you change your mindset. The mindset is like a box where your beliefs and ideas are created. It gives you the power to trust yourself and the key to success.

Let me give you an example. Think about any successful athlete.

Have they always been successful? No.

Have they ever struggled in their career? Yes.

Have they ever failed? Yes.

But, even when they had doubts (we all have them at times), they behaved and thought like athletes. They trained hard, ate healthily, avoided drinking alcohol, and looked after their bodies as much as possible, as most athletes do.

Similarly to athletes, maintaining a sugar-free life requires commitment. We will discuss this in the next section, but think of who you are before you get there.

How do you identify yourself?

Are you a recovered sugar-free addict who can slip into old habits anytime, or are you someone who values a healthy lifestyle and chooses to live a sugar-free life? Who would you rather be? More importantly, why do you want to be that person?

Making a Long-Term Commitment

Living healthily is a big commitment, and maintaining a sugar-free diet is an essential part of that commitment. It's a lifestyle that requires you to change your behaviour, and it's not something you do for a limited time.

Most people struggle with changing their behaviours, and my clients find it difficult too. But when they start experiencing positive results — feeling more energised, having a clearer mind and younger-looking skin — they can see the value in what they are doing and feel encouraged to continue with their commitment.

But how can you hold yourself accountable to carry on when things get tough, you may ask? That is a great question.

Lack of accountability destroys many dreams. Personal responsibility plays a significant role in a person's success.

I recommend that you keep revisiting your *why*. Only then, you'll be able to stay committed to your decisions and carry on when things get difficult.

Do you remember your *why* from Day One? Your commitment to your goal will be only as good as your *why*.

We all have good and bad days. On good days, we feel happy, excited, grateful and inspired. But on bad days, we might feel lonely, sad, anxious or stressed.

On good days, the commitment to taking positive actions might be high. But on bad days, the struggle is real.

What can you do when you are feeling discouraged and low? How do you find motivation? How do you find dedication? Here are a few suggestions:

- *Write or print out your pledge to give up sugar*: Write it in your diary, or print it out and put it on the fridge door, the bedroom wall, or the bathroom mirror...

wherever is convenient for you. The pledge must include why you are doing it, and it needs to be something you feel strongly about. Do you do it because you want to be healthy in your old age and see your children or grandchildren growing up? This is a great reason to have. Make sure you find something that resonates with you and that you feel strongly about and proud of when visualising your success. Put your pledge where you can see it daily, and you will be reminded why you need to carry on.

- *Keep a food diary and note your successes and failures*: There's no need to beat yourself up if you do slip up — but having to write it down will remind you to try harder in the future.

- *Tell your family and close friends what you're doing*: Speak to people close to you and ask them to remind you if you're ever tempted to slip. You may find it great encouragement to see your family and friends cheering for and supporting you. At the same time, the embarrassment of letting down people around you could be a powerful motive to stick to your commitment.

- *Search through social media for mutual support groups*: Whether these focus on a sugar-free diet or, more generally, on healthy eating, they offer encouragement and advice. Group support could be very powerful. Don't ever underestimate it!

- *Work with a health and diet professional*: They'll encourage you to stick to your sugar-free diet and help you deal with any problems that might arise in the short-term. They'll also be able to advise you about more general aspects of your diet.

If you'd like to find out how I can help you to achieve your goals and improve your well-being, feel free to contact me. I'd love to help. Here's the link for your convenience: www.silvanahealthandnutrition.com/booking/. I am always pleased to support the readers of my books and offer them my knowledge and expertise to improve their health, be more in tune with their bodies, and be in charge of their well-being.

Day Ten Task: Write a Sugar-Free Agreement with Yourself

Now, I'm challenging you to sign the agreement with yourself about committing to a sugar-free life after you've finished the 10 Day programme. This is vital for your success.

When writing the contract, be positive, encouraging, and compassionate about your needs.

Here is an example of your sugar-free contract (fill out the dots in the text):

Dear Me, I promise myself that I'll commit to continuing with my new behaviour and not go back to eating sugar. I want to live a sugar-free life because…. . And if I occasionally slip back into my old habits, I will …. . It is essential that I take care of my body because ….. . A sugar-free life will help me to ….. . (Add any text that applies to you) ….. .

Bonus Chapter

30 Anti-Inflammatory Recipes

In this bonus chapter of the book, I will share with you 30 sugar-free recipes for breakfast, lunch, dinner, and desserts.

And that's not all.

I often see people struggling when preparing sugar-free meals, so I decided to give you tips on meal planning that will provide you with the necessary tools to effortlessly create healthy meal plans in the future. This will allow you to enjoy good health for many years from now.

Meal Planning

One of the valuable strategies to keep yourself sugar-free in the long-term is to make weekly meal plans — at least until planning a healthy, sugar-free meal becomes second nature.

Here are a few suggestions on how to do this:

1. Identify Your Ingredients

- Brainstorm your favourite food ingredients — anything you might want to include in a meal or a snack. These might be simple foods, like any vegetables, meat or fish, or even packaged produce that you like eating.

- The next step is to go through each item and identify whether or not it is sugar-free. Use the knowledge you gained through reading this book, and do additional research if necessary. Don't forget that "sugar-free" doesn't always mean the product is free from sugar. Research is key!

- You can also make a "reserve list" of foods with added sugar in low quantities. These are still best avoided for now while you're still vulnerable to sugar cravings, but you may be able to add them later.

- When you make a list of sugar-free ingredients for your meals, see if you can identify which nutrients contain proteins, healthy carbs and healthy fats. This will help you prepare balanced meals.

2. Create a Database of Meals

- Once you have a list of your favourite ingredients, it is time to turn them into a range of meals, which might simply be combinations of simple foods or more elaborate recipes. You can create your own recipes or search through the recipes I have included in this book. You will find plenty of delicious sugar-free recipes in the next section of this book, but learning to create the recipes from scratch or searching online will give you a range of ideas for making your meal plans varied and exciting, which is crucial for the long-term success of your sugar-free diet.

- Create a substantial list of meals suitable for breakfast, lunch, and dinner, and a list of sugar-free snacks. You can continue adding to this list when you find new ideas.

- Check each meal for nutritional balance. Ensure you're getting a good balance of proteins, fibre, natural sugar, and unsaturated fat, and a wide selection of vitamins and minerals. "Eat the rainbow" is an excellent guideline to follow.

3. Draw up a Weekly Meal Plan

- Go through your list of meals and make up a plan for the next seven days, including breakfast, lunch, dinner, and snacks. Make sure your meals include a variety of essential nutrients.
- Finally, think about your schedule for each day. If you are making a dinner that will take an hour to prepare and you're rushing to go out, it'll tempt you to abandon the plan and reach for something at random — which may or may not be sugar-free.
- Now, you have a meal plan for the week. I want to encourage you to do a weekly meal plan until reaching for sugar-free foods becomes second nature.

In the rest of this book, you'll find recipes to help you prepare your menu plan. Check online for more great ideas to make your meals more varied and exciting.

Make sure you eat the rainbow to give your body what it needs.

Enjoy the recipes, and I wish you all the best in continuing your sugar-free life.

Anti-Inflammatory Breakfast Recipes

Tomato Poached Eggs [21]

Servings: 4

Nutrition: calories 195, protein 6g, carbohydrates 19g, fibre 4g, fat 3.5g

Ingredients:

- 1 celery stick, chopped
- 2 shallots, chopped
- 60ml extra virgin olive oil
- 2 cloves of garlic, chopped
- 4 eggs
- 1 jar of passata (700g)
- ½ bunch flat-leaf parsley, chopped
- 1 long red chilli, chopped

Method:

1. Take a pan and heat over a medium temperature
2. Add the oil and allow to warm up, before adding the shallots, garlic, chilli, parsley, and celery
3. Cook for 3 minutes
4. Pour the passata into the pan and 125ml of water
5. Allow to boil and then reduce the heat to simmer, leaving for 15 minutes to reduce
6. Make 4 holes in the mixture
7. Crack one egg into each hole
8. Cook for 5 minutes to your liking
9. Decorate with extra parsley leaves and serve while warm

Overnight Oats [22]

Servings: 4

Nutrition: calories 215, protein 9g, carbohydrates 33g, fibre 4g, fat 5g

Ingredients:

- 64g oats
- 235ml almond milk
- 0.25 tsp cinnamon
- 1 tsp almond, crushed
- 1 tsp hemp seeds

Method:

1. Take a small bowl and add your oats
2. Pour the almond milk over the oats, soaking completely
3. Sprinkle the cinnamon, almond and hemp seeds over the oats and combine mix
4. Leave in the refrigerator overnight

Cream Cheese & Smoked Salmon Omelette [23]

Servings: 2

Nutrition: calories 254, protein 16.8g, carbohydrates 2.7g, fibre 0.3g, fat 12g

Ingredients:

- 1 tsp butter
- 2 large eggs
- 2 tbsp smoked salmon, chopped

- 1 tbsp softened cream cheese
- Quarter of red onion, chopped
- 1.5 tsp fresh dill, chopped
- 1 tsp water
- Salt and pepper to garnish

Method:

1. Take a small mixing bowl and add eggs, water, and a little salt and pepper, combining well
2. Take a small frying pan and add the butter over medium to low heat
3. Add the egg to the pan and cook for a minute
4. Add cheese, dill, finely chopped onion, and salmon over one half of the cooking omelette
5. Allow to cook for 3 minutes, until all the egg is cooked
6. Flip the empty side of the omelette over the filled side and cook for a further minute
7. Flip the omelette over and continue to cook for another minute
8. Transfer to your serving plate

Green Almond Milk Smoothie [24]

Servings: 2

Nutrition: calories 343, protein 5.9g, carbohydrates 54g, fibre 12.1g, fat 3g

Ingredients:

- 236ml vanilla almond milk
- 1 ripe banana
- 1 tbsp chia seeds
- Quarter of an avocado, peeled and chopped
- 125g baby kale

- A handful of ice cubes

Method:

1. Add all the ingredients to your blender, except for the ice cubes
2. Blend on a high speed until everything is smooth and creamy
3. Add the ice cubes and blend for another minute
4. Pour into serving glasses

Egg & Broccoli [25]

Servings: 4

Nutrition: calories 215, protein 9g, carbohydrates 33g, fibre 4g, fat 5g

Ingredients:

- 1 broccoli, chopped
- 1 egg
- 1 sliced red onion
- 1 tsp extra virgin olive oil

Method:

1. Take a medium frying pan and add the oil over medium heat
2. Place the broccoli and onion in the pan and cook until wilted
3. Transfer the broccoli and onion onto a plate
4. Crack the egg into the pan and cook to your liking
5. Serve the egg on top of the broccoli and onion mixture

Mock Hash Browns [26]

Servings: 4

Nutrition: calories 200, protein 3g, carbohydrates 35g, fibre 3g, fat 6g

Ingredients:

- 3 tbsp canola oil
- 1 large onion, grated
- 4 potatoes, grated
- 1 tsp salt
- 0.25 tsp garlic powder
- 0.25 tsp pepper

Method:

1. Take a large skillet pan and add the oil, over medium to high heat
2. Take a bowl and combine the onion, potatoes, garlic powder, salt, and pepper
3. Form patties with the mixture and cook in the pan on each side for 7 minutes

Egg & Salsa Verde Salad [27]

Servings: 1

Nutrition: calories 527, protein 16g, carbohydrates 37g, fibre 13g, fat 11g

Ingredients:

- 1 tbsp extra virgin olive oil, plus an extra 1 tsp
- 8 blue corn tortilla chips, crumbled

- 1 egg
- Quarter of a sliced avocado
- 250g salad greens
- 3 tbsp salsa verde
- Half a can of rinsed red kidney beans
- 2 tbsp coriander, chopped

Method:

1. Take a small bowl and combine the 1 tbs of olive oil, coriander, and salsa
2. Transfer half the mixture into a bowl and toss with the salad greens, retaining the other half
3. Add the crumbled tortilla chips, avocado, and kidney beans on top of the salad greens
4. Take a small frying pan and add the rest of the oil
5. Fry the egg to your liking and once cooked, transfer on top of the salad
6. Drizzle the rest of the vinaigrette over the top of the salad before serving

Trout & Kale Breakfast Bowl [28]

Servings: 1

Nutrition: calories 275, protein 10g, carbohydrates 9.4g, fibre 4.5g, fat 23g

Ingredients:

- 1 tbsp olive oil
- 2 tsp red wine vinegar
- 1 tsp minced garlic
- 31g flaked smoked trout
- 375g baby kale
- Quarter of a chopped red onion

- Quarter of a diced avocado
- Salt and pepper for seasoning

Method:

1. Add the garlic and a little salt into a small bowl and use a fork to mash them down into a paste
2. Take another bowl and add the oil, vinegar, pepper and garlic paste, mixing well
3. Add the kale to the bowl and coat well
4. Take a serving bowl and add the trout, red onion, and avocado
5. Top with the kale before serving

Anti-Inflammatory Lunch Recipes

Quinoa & Salmon Salad [29]

Servings: 4

Nutrition: calories 464, protein 33g, carbohydrates 19g, fibre 2.5g, fat 4g

Ingredients:

- 3 tbsp olive oil, plus an extra 2 tbsp for cooking
- 2 tbsp balsamic vinegar
- 1 minced garlic clove
- 1 tsp Dijon mustard
- 450g skinned wild salmon
- 272g cooked quinoa (set aside to cool)
- 544g rocket/arugula
- Half an onion, chopped
- Half a tomato, chopped
- Salt and pepper for seasoning

Method:

1. Take a small mixing bowl and combine the balsamic vinegar, 3 tbs olive oil, garlic, Dijon mustard and a little salt and pepper to taste. Set the mixture to one side
2. Take a large bowl and add the quinoa, rocket/arugula, tomato, onion, and the balsamic mixture. Season and combine well
3. Take your salmon fillets and season well
4. Take a large skillet and add 2 tbs olive oil, over medium heat
5. Cook the salmon on the skin side first for around 4 minutes and then turn over and cook until completely done
6. Place to one side to cool
7. Once cooled, use a fork to flake the salmon and add to the salad bowl, mixing well before serving

Lentil Soup With a Kick [30]

Servings: 6

Nutrition: calories 260, protein 8g, carbohydrates 24g, fibre 8g, fat 16g

Ingredients:

- 1.5 tbsp extra virgin olive oil
- 1 can of diced tomatoes
- 1 can of coconut milk
- 140g baby spinach
- 140g red lentils, uncooked and rinsed
- 875ml vegetable broth
- 2 garlic cloves, minced
- 1 large onion, chopped
- 1.5 tsp ground cumin

- 2 tsp ground turmeric
- 0.25 tsp ground cardamom
- 0.5 tsp cinnamon
- 0.5 tsp red pepper flakes
- 2 tsp lime juice
- Salt and pepper to taste

Method:

1. Take a large soup pot and add the oil, garlic, onion, and a little salt
2. Using medium heat, cook for 5 minutes, stirring occasionally, until the onion is soft
3. Add the cardamom, cumin, cinnamon, and turmeric, and cook for another minute
4. Add the can of tomatoes, coconut milk, vegetable broth, red lentils, red pepper flakes, and season with salt and pepper, combining well
5. Turn the heat up and bring the contents to a boil, then reduce to a simmer and leave to cook uncovered for around 20 minutes
6. Remove from the heat and add the spinach, stirring until it wilts
7. Add the lime juice and a little more seasoning if required

Lunchtime Tuna Salad [31]

Servings: 6

Nutrition: calories 147, protein 8g, carbohydrates 12g, fibre 3.4g, fat 8.8g

Ingredients:

- 2 cans of tuna, drained

- 1 can of sun-dried tomatoes, chopped
- 1 chopped cucumber
- 1 small red onion, diced
- 125g roasted red peppers, chopped
- 2 tsp capers
- Half an avocado, diced
- 41g chopped parsley
- 2 tbsp red wine vinegar
- 2 tbsp olive oil
- 1 tsp dried oregano
- 1 tsp lemon juice
- 1 tsp dried parsley
- Salt and pepper for seasoning

Method:

1. Take a large bowl and mix the tuna, sun-dried tomatoes, cucumber, red onion, red peppers, capers, avocado, and chopped parsley
2. Take a small bowl and mix the red wine vinegar, olive oil, dried oregano, lemon juice, dried parsley and a little salt and pepper
3. Pour the dressing over the salad ingredients and toss to coat well
4. Transfer to serving plates

Red Lentil & Tomato Pasta [32]

Servings: 6

Nutrition: calories 300, protein 8g, carbohydrates 16g, fibre 14g, fat 17.5g

Ingredients:

- 60ml extra virgin olive oil

- 1 can of fire-roasted tomatoes
- 62g sun-dried tomatoes, chopped
- 2 handfuls of baby spinach
- 6 cloves of garlic, minced
- 1 onion, chopped
- 2 tsp ground turmeric
- 1 tbsp dried basil
- 1 tbsp dried oregano
- 1 tbsp apple cider vinegar
- 225g red lentil pasta

Method:

1. Take a large cooking pot and add the oil, and heat over a medium temperature
2. Add the onion and allow to cook for 5-10 minutes, until softened
3. Add the oregano, basil, turmeric, garlic, and a little salt and pepper, combining and cooking for another minute
4. Add the canned tomatoes and use the fork to crush them down a little
5. Add the vinegar and sun-dried tomatoes and stir
6. Allow to simmer for 15 minutes
7. Add the spinach and cook for another 5 minutes
8. Take another pot and cook the pasta to your liking, draining once cooked
9. Divide the pasta between your bowls and add a large spoonful of the sauce on top

Coconut Chickpea Curry [33]

Servings: 4

Nutrition: calories 665, protein 26g, carbohydrates 80g, fibre 14g, fat 31g

Ingredients:

- 1 tbsp extra virgin olive oil
- 1 can of coconut milk
- 1 can of chickpeas
- 3 tbsp red curry paste
- 3 minced garlic cloves
- 1 sliced red bell pepper
- 1 sliced red onion
- 1 small cauliflower, cut into small florets
- 1 lime, cut into halves
- 187g frozen peas
- 31g fresh coriander, chopped
- 4 chopped spring onions
- 1 tsp ground coriander
- 1 tbsp minced fresh ginger
- 2 tsp chilli powder
- Salt and pepper to taste

Method:

1. Take a large pan and add the olive oil, heating over a medium temperature
2. Add the pepper and onion and cook for 5 minutes
3. Add the garlic and ginger and cook for another minute
4. Add the cauliflower and make sure everything is coated and combined
5. Add the coriander, chilli powder, and red curry paste, cooking for another minute
6. Add the coconut milk and stir, bringing to a simmer
7. Cover the pan and allow to simmer for 10 minutes
8. Take the lid off the pan and add the lime juice, mixing well
9. Add the frozen peas, chickpeas, salt, and pepper and combine

10. Allow the mixture to simmer for 10 minutes
11. Add to serving bowls and garnish with coriander and spring onions

Turkey Taco Bowls [34]

Servings: 2

Nutrition: calories 370, protein 29g, carbohydrates 52g, fibre 5g, fat 7g

Ingredients:

- 93g uncooked brown rice
- 1 lime
- 350g ground turkey
- 2 tbsp taco seasoning
- 150ml water
- 10 cherry tomatoes, halved
- 1 chopped jalapeño pepper
- Quarter a chopped red onion
- The juice and zest of half a lime
- Salt and pepper for seasoning
- 62g grated mozzarella

Method:

1. Take the brown rice and cook according to the instructions on the packet
2. Add the zest from the lime and a little salt to the water as the rice is cooking and place to one side to cool
3. Take a medium frying pan and cook the turkey over medium heat for 10 minutes
4. Add the taco seasoning and combine well
5. Add the water and stir well, allowing to simmer for a few minutes

6. Remove the pan from the heat and allow it to cool
7. Take a bowl and add the cherry tomatoes, jalapeño, and red onion. Mix it well
8. Serve the turkey over the salsa with the mozzarella sprinkled on top

Zesty Chicken Wraps [35]

Servings: 4

Nutrition: calories 612, protein 32g, carbohydrates 48g, fibre 29g, fat 22g

Ingredients:

- 1.5 tsp olive oil plus 1 tbsp extra
- 2 chicken breasts with the bone left in
- 4 whole wheat tortilla wraps
- 62g hummus
- 62g feta cheese
- 4 tbsp kalamata olives
- 1 tbsp red wine vinegar
- 300g romaine, chopped
- 1 cucumber, chopped
- 1 small red onion, chopped
- 5 cherry tomatoes, sliced
- 1 tsp dried oregano
- 1 tsp lemon pepper
- 1 tsp garlic powder

Method:

1. Preheat the oven to 200C and prepare a baking sheet with baking parchment
2. Place the chicken onto the baking tray

3. In a small bowl, combine the oregano, lemon pepper, garlic powder, salt and pepper
4. Rub the spice mixture over the chicken breasts evenly
5. Drizzle the chicken with 1.5 tsp of olive oil
6. Cook in the oven for 40 minutes, until the chicken is completely cooked
7. Take a large bowl and add the romaine, tomatoes, red onion, olives, cucumber and feta cheese, combining well
8. Drizzle the remaining olive oil and vinegar over the top with a little fresh lemon juice, combining well
9. Assemble the wrap by taking one tortilla at a time, adding some of the chicken and a large spoonful of the salad. Wrap up the edges and repeat with the other tortillas

Anti-Inflammatory Dinner Recipes

Spinach & Chickpea Stew [36]

Servings: 6

Nutrition: calories 401, protein 32g, carbohydrates 41g, fibre 13g, fat 13g

Ingredients:

- 1 tbsp olive oil
- 2 cans of chickpeas, rinsed
- 340g ground turkey
- 1 chopped onion
- 2 chopped carrots
- 3 tbsp tomato paste
- 225g spinach
- 950ml chicken broth

- 4 garlic cloves, minced
- 0.5 tsp dried oregano
- 0.5 tsp crushed red pepper
- 0.5 tsp crushed fennel seeds
- Salt and pepper to taste

Method:

1. Take a mixing bowl and add one can of chickpeas. Use a fork to mash into a smooth mixture
2. Take a large cooking pot and add the olive oil over medium to high heat
3. Add the turkey and use a wooden spoon to break it up into small pieces
4. Add the fennel seeds, oregano, and red pepper, and cook for around 4 minutes
5. Add the carrots, onion and garlic and cook for another 4 minutes
6. Add the tomato paste and mix well, cooking for a further minute
7. Add the chicken broth and stir
8. Add the mashed chickpeas and the remaining can of chickpeas with a little salt and pepper
9. Mix well and cover the pan, bringing to the boil
10. Reduce the heat and leave the lid on, cooking at a simmer for 10 minutes
11. Add the spinach to the pan and turn the heat up a little
12. Cook for two minutes, and serve

Chicken & Artichoke Casserole [37]

Servings: 4

Nutrition: calories 396, protein 47g, carbohydrates 19g, fibre 6g, fat 14g

Ingredients:

- 1 tbsp olive oil
- 450g skinless chicken breasts, cut into chunks
- 1 can of artichoke hearts, chopped
- 2 minced garlic cloves
- 500g cauliflower rice
- 118ml chicken broth
- 375g spinach, chopped
- 350ml full-fat Greek yoghurt
- 125g grated mozzarella cheese
- Salt and pepper to taste

Method:

1. Preheat the oven to 190C
2. Take a baking dish and spray with cooking spray
3. Take a large cooking pot and add the oil over a medium heat
4. Add the chicken and season, stirring and cooking for 5 minutes
5. Add the garlic, stir and cook for a further minute
6. Add the broth and the artichoke and mix well once more, cooking for another 4 minutes
7. Take the pot from the heat and add the cauliflower rice, stirring well
8. Add the spinach, yoghurt, and half the mozzarella, mix once more
9. Place the mixture into your baking dish and add the rest of the cheese over the top
10. Cook in the oven for 20 minutes
11. Cool for 5 minutes before serving

Sweet Potato & Quinoa Chilli [38]

Servings: 6

Nutrition: calories 346, protein 12g, carbohydrates 63g, fibre 11g, fat 6g

Ingredients:

- 1 tbsp olive oil
- 950ml vegetable broth
- 125g uncooked white quinoa
- 1 can of pinto beans, rinsed
- 1 can of diced tomatoes
- 2 peeled sweet potatoes, cut into small chunks
- 2 diced poblano peppers
- 1 diced onion
- 4 chopped garlic cloves
- 1 can of diced green chillis
- 470ml water
- 1 tbsp chilli powder
- 2 tsp ground cumin
- Salt and pepper for seasoning

Method:

1. Take a large cooking pot and add the oil over medium to high heat
2. Cook the sweet potatoes until soft, for around 8 minutes and add the poblanos and the onion and cook for another 3 minutes
3. Add the chilli powder, garlic, and cumin, stirring and cooking for another 30 seconds
4. Add the tomatoes, green chillies, and the broth, mix well and add half the water, stirring once more

5. Cover the pan over and turn the heat up, bringing the pan to the boil
6. Add the beans, quinoa, and a little seasoning, stirring again
7. Reduce the heat to medium and cover the pan over, allowing it to simmer
8. Cook for 15 minutes, and then add the other half of the water during the last 5 minutes, combining well
9. Season to your taste

Spinach & Mushroom Pasta [39]

Serving: 4

Nutrition: calories 276, protein 10g, carbohydrates 35g, fibre 5g, fat 14g

Ingredients:

- 4 tbsp olive oil
- 226g wholewheat fettuccine pasta
- 375g baby spinach
- 700g sliced cremini mushrooms
- 2 tsp Worcestershire sauce
- 6 tbsp unsalted, roasted pistachios, chopped
- 3 tbsp balsamic vinegar
- 2 sliced garlic cloves
- 31g fresh basil, chopped
- Salt and pepper to season

Method:

1. Cook the pasta according to the packet instructions
2. Once cooked, drain and keep a quarter of the cooking water to one side

3. Take a large frying pan and add 2 tbsp of the oil over medium to high heat
4. Cook the mushrooms for 10 minutes, stirring occasionally
5. Add the garlic and combine, cooking for 1 minute
6. Add the spinach and stir constantly for another minute
7. Turn the heat down to medium to low and add the balsamic vinegar, salt, pepper, the rest of the oil, and Worcestershire sauce. Combine well
8. Add the pasta and toss to fully coat
9. Add the rest of the cooking water and stir
10. Add the basil and pistachios just before serving

Quinoa & Beet Larb [40]

Servings: 4

Nutrition: calories 279, protein 8.2g, carbohydrates 42g, fibre 7g, fat 9.6g

Ingredients:

- 2 tbsp canola oil
- 450g peeled red beets, chopped
- 1 cabbage, shredded
- 1 cucumber, sliced
- 1 carrot, sliced
- 125g mint leaves
- 95g black rice
- 95g quinoa
- 150ml lime juice
- 2 tbsp fish sauce
- 31g spring onions, chopped
- 2 tbsp fresh coriander, chopped
- 0.25 tsp crushed red pepper

- 350ml water, plus another 2 tbsp extra

Method:

1. Take a large frying pan and add the rice, toasting for 5 minutes, stirring regularly
2. Use a mortar and pestle to grind the rice down to a powder and place to one side
3. Take a medium saucepan and add the quinoa and 350ml of water
4. Bring the pan to the boil and then reduce down to a low simmer, cooking for 20 minutes, until the water has absorbed
5. Take a small bowl and add the rest of the water, spring onions, lime juice, coriander, crushed red pepper, and the fish sauce, combining well
6. Take another skillet and add the oil over medium to high heat
7. Cook the beet, stirring occasionally, for around 4 minutes
8. Add half the combined mixture from the bowl and the ground rice, stirring well.
9. Cook for 2 minutes
10. Divide the quinoa between 4 serving bowls and top with the beet mixture, cucumber, cabbage, carrot, and herbs.
11. If there is any sauce left, drizzle over the top and garnish with mint

Salty Chicken With Brussels Sprouts [41]

Servings: 4

Nutrition: calories 387, protein 35g, carbohydrates 19g, fibre 6g, fat 18g

Ingredients:

- 3 tbsp olive oil
- 680g chicken breasts with the skin and bone left on
- 680g Brussels sprouts, cut into halves
- 2 red onions, cut into wedges
- 6 tbsp malt vinegar
- 0.5 tsp dried dill
- 0.5 tsp garlic powder
- 0.5 tsp onion powder
- Salt and pepper for seasoning

Method:

1. Preheat your oven to 230C
2. Take the chicken breasts and cut them into four portions
3. Brush the chicken with 1 tbs of the oil and season
4. Take a large bowl and add the Brussels sprouts with the onions, the rest of the oil and a little salt and pepper
5. Place the chicken and vegetables onto a baking tray
6. Put in the oven and cook for 25 minutes, making sure the chicken is cooked through
7. Take a microwave-safe bowl and add the garlic powder, dill, onion powder, and vinegar with a little salt and combine well
8. Place in the microwave on high for 30 seconds
9. Remove the chicken tray from the oven and drizzle the mixture over the contents
10. Place back in the oven for another 5 minutes

Hearty Slow Cooker Stew [42]

Servings: 4

Nutrition: calories 191, protein 5.7g, carbohydrates 22g, fibre 5.6g, fat 7.8g

Ingredients:

- 3 tbsp olive oil
- 700ml vegetable broth
- 2 can of fire roasted, diced tomatoes
- 1 chopped carrot
- 1 chopped onion
- 4 minced garlic cloves
- 1 bunch of chopped kale
- 1 can of chickpeas
- 1 tbsp lemon juice
- 1 tsp dried oregano
- 0.5 tsp crushed red pepper
- Salt and pepper for seasoning

Method:

1. Add the broth, tomatoes, carrot, onion, crushed red pepper, garlic, oregano, salt and pepper into your slow cooker
2. Cover and cook for 6 hours on a low setting
3. After 5.5 hours have passed, take 60ml of the cooking water from the slow cooker and place it into a separate small mixing bowl
4. Add 2 tbs of the chickpeas and use a fork to mash them down
5. Add the mixture back to the slow cooker along with the lemon juice, kale and the rest of the chickpeas from the can
6. Stir well and cover back over to cook for another 30 minutes

Avocado & Salmon Dinner Bowls [43]

Servings: 2

Nutrition: calories 442, protein 29g, carbohydrates 34g, fibre 7g, fat 21g

Ingredients:

- 450g frozen wild salmon, cut into cubes
- 2 tsp toasted sesame oil
- 3 tbsp tamari
- 31g caviar
- Pinch of cayenne pepper
- 1 diced avocado
- 62g sliced spring onions
- 62g sliced onion
- 62g chopped coriander
- 2 tbsp rice vinegar
- 2 tbsp olive oil
- 250g short grain brown rice, cooked
- 250g arugula or watercress
- 1 tbsp Dijon mustard

Method:

1. Take a medium mixing bowl and add the avocado, spring onions, coriander, salmon, caviar, cayenne pepper, tamari, and sesame oil, mixing well
2. Take a large bowl and add the arugula or watercress with the rice
3. In a small bowl, mix the Dijon and olive oil, before adding to the rice bowl
4. Serve with the salad mixture over the top

Anti-Inflammatory Dessert Recipes

Fruity Sorbet [44]

Servings: 4

Nutrition: calories 170, protein 3g, carbohydrates 43g, fibre 3g, fat 1g

Ingredients:

- 1 medium watermelon

Method:

1. Take a baking sheet
2. Place the cubes of watermelon on the baking sheet in one layer
3. Place the baking sheet into the freezer for around 2 hours; after that time the watermelon should be totally frozen
4. Place the watermelon into a blender and mix until smooth
5. Transfer the blended watermelon into a deep baking dish or a loaf tin and press down so you can place more inside
6. Keep blending the rest of the watermelon and transferring it to the same dish/tin
7. Place it in the freezer for around 1.5 hours, or until you can easily scoop the consistency of sorbet

Date and Chocolate Sugar-Free Pudding [45]

Servings: 8

Nutrition: calories 280, protein 8g, carbohydrates 32g, fibre 3g, fat 5g

Ingredients:

- 150g buckwheat flour
- 375g pitted, fresh dates
- 300g almond meal
- 1.5 tsp bicarbonate of soda
- 300ml buttermilk
- 35g raw cacao powder
- 1 vanilla bean
- 225g solidified coconut oil
- 150g sugar-free dark chocolate, chopped
- 6 beaten eggs

For vanilla and coconut sauce, use the following ingredients:

- 800ml coconut milk
- 200g pitted, fresh dates
- 2 vanilla beans

Method:

1. Preheat the oven to 180C
2. Take a 2.5 litre baking dish and grease liberally
3. Place 200g of dates into a bowl and add 750ml of boiling water over the top
4. Allow to sit for 10 minutes
5. After 10 minutes have passed, drain and chop the dates
6. In a large bowl, add the chopped dates with other ingredients and stir. Combine well
7. Transfer the mixture to the baking dish, distributing evenly and smoothing out the top

8. Place in the oven and cook for 50 minutes to 1 hour
9. In the meantime, make the vanilla and coconut sauce. Take the saucepan and combine all ingredients. Stir over high heat and allow the mixture to simmer. Then remove from the heat
10. Place it into a blender and blend until you get a smooth mixture
11. Set aside for 10 minutes
12. Once the cake has cooked, poke a few holes from top to bottom using a knife and pour some of the sauce over the hot cake, allowing it to soak in
13. The rest of the sauce can be served on the side

Banana Pancakes [46]

Servings: 2

Nutrition: calories 243, protein 9g, carbohydrates 15g, fibre 4g, fat 15g

Ingredients:

- 1 large banana
- 2 eggs
- 1 tsp coconut oil
- 125g raspberries
- 25g roughly chopped pecan

Method:

1. Mash the banana in the bowl using the fork
2. Add two eggs and mix it all thoroughly
3. Add 1 tsp coconut oil to a hot frying pan
4. Fry each side of the pancake for approximately 1 minute then put it on the plate
5. Top the pancakes with pecans and raspberries

Apple & Cinnamon Crunch [47]

Servings: 6

Nutrition: calories 65, protein 3g, carbohydrates 18g, fibre 5g, fat 5g

Ingredients:

- 3 large apples
- 0.75 tsp ground cinnamon

Method:

1. Preheat your oven to 100C and arrange the racks in the top and bottom oven
2. Take two baking sheets and prepare them with baking parchment
3. Core the apples and then cut into rounds
4. Place the apple rounds onto the baking sheets in an even layer
5. Sprinkle the cinnamon over the top
6. Bake in the oven for 1 hour
7. After an hour, switch the trays around, so the one that was on the top is now in the bottom tray and vice versa
8. Cook for another hour
9. Allow the apple crisps to cool completely before eating

Date Milkshake [48]

Servings: 1

Nutrition: calories 333, protein 5g, carbohydrates 21g, fibre 3g, fat 3g

Ingredients:

- 4 pitted dates
- 2 frozen bananas
- 2 tbsp chia seeds
- 2 tbsp unsweetened almond milk
- 0.5 tsp cinnamon
- 2 tbsp sugar-free peanut butter

Method:

1. Take a blender and add all the ingredients inside
2. Blend for 1-2 minutes, until you achieve a smooth and thick consistency
3. Pour into a serving glass and enjoy immediately

Decadent Hot Chocolate [49]

Servings: 2

Nutrition: calories 253, protein 3g, carbohydrates 7g, fibre 4g, fat 8g

Ingredients:

- 470ml coconut milk (you can also use almond milk as an alternative)
- 1 tbsp coconut oil
- 2 tbsp cacao
- 1 tsp maca powder
- 0.25 tsp ground turmeric
- 0.5 tsp ground cinnamon

Method:

1. Take a medium saucepan and add the milk over medium heat, bringing it to the boil

2. Turn the heat down and allow it to simmer before adding the cacao and stir well
3. Add the cinnamon, turmeric, and maca powder and combine
4. Add the coconut oil and use a whisk to break up. The mixture should be thick at this point
5. Pour into cups and serve

Slow Rice Pudding [50]

Servings: 6

Nutrition: calories 200, protein 8g, carbohydrates 32g, fibre 1g, fat 4g

Ingredients:

- 200g wholegrain rice
- 1 litre of semi-skimmed milk
- 1 tsp butter
- 1 tsp cinnamon
- A few flaked almonds to serve

Method:

1. Grease the inside of your slow cooker
2. Take a medium saucepan and heat up the milk until it starts to gently simmer
3. Place in the slow cooker
4. Add the rice and mix
5. Add a little cinnamon and combine
6. Cook on a high setting for 2.5 hours, stirring a couple of times throughout
7. Serve with flaked almonds on the top

I wrote this book with the intention of helping you break the sugar habit and improve your relationship with food so that you can lead a healthier and happier life. I'd love to know if I succeeded. Let me know how you're getting on.

Conclusion

So here you are, at the end of your 10 Day Sugar Detox Challenge. But, as I said in the final chapter, this isn't the end of the process by any means. It's time to make up your mind about what you're going to do now — and what you've learned in this book will give you the tools you'll need.

You now understand how damaging added sugar (also called processed sugar or free sugar) can be to both your physical and mental health. It can create issues from heart disease, abdominal fat and increased risk of type 2 diabetes to stress and depression. And you also know why it's so hard to give sugar up. All this time, you've been addicted to a substance that acts much like a drug.

That's because your body still thinks you're a primitive human, hunting and avoiding being mauled by dangerous beasts. In this respect, it quite rightly encourages you to stock up on sugar to give you extra energy whenever you're stressed. The problem is that today's stresses don't usually need this energy, so it's left to damage your body and your brain — but despite the damage sugar is causing, your brain craves more of it.

Sugar would be easier to avoid, of course, if it wasn't around us everywhere. Our primitive ancestors got their sugar mainly from natural sources, such as fruit and vegetables, which the body can process correctly for the energy it needs. Not only is most of the sugar we encounter today unhealthy added sugar, but it can be found in almost all processed foods and drinks. Even if you examine the ingredients list carefully, it's often included under a misleading name.

So, between the cravings your brain produces and temptations everywhere, it isn't easy to give up sugar — but it is possible. I've given you various strategies in this book, such as shopping carefully, sugar-proofing your home and office, and identifying how to eat out safely. I've also explained how to identify if you're eating emotionally, how to use mindfulness to counteract this, and how to deal with sugar cravings. In the final chapter, you received a variety of strategies to continue living sugar-free.

And have you completed all the tasks? If you've skipped any, I'd strongly suggest you go back and complete them because each one of them is going to help you carry on with your sugar-free life. The Workbook is designed to help you with this process.

If you have done them all, you'll know what your personal motivation is for giving up sugar — and that's essential for sticking to your plan. You'll also have learned to identify which foods and drinks contain added sugar and which don't. You should have cleared out sugary foods from your kitchen, and identified where you can safely eat out.

You were also encouraged to identify your own sugar triggers and practice mindful eating to help you fight them, as well as overcoming your sugar cravings. Finally, you learned how to create weekly meal plans so you can enjoy improved health.

You've probably been through a rough ten days dealing with the withdrawal symptoms of giving up sugar. Besides battling the cravings, you may have suffered from headaches, brain fog, mood swings, digestion problems and even skin irritations.

Hopefully, these have cleared up by now, or they'll be clearing up over the next few days. You'll still be experiencing cravings for a while, but they should get easier to resist over the coming weeks. And, as your body gradually detoxes from your sugar habit, you'll find you have more energy, sharper thinking and generally feel better than you have in a long time.

You'll feel no desire to return to the old mood swings and general poor health — so don't let yourself forget that giving up sugar made the difference.

So what are you going to do now? At the end of the final chapter, I challenged you to make a long-term commitment to continue living sugar-free. Sticking to a commitment is easier when you not only have support, but also someone who can hold you sensitively but firmly to account. There are various options for this, but the surest method would be to let me help you.

So why me?

Well, besides my training and experience in counselling, psychology, and nutrition, and working with clients for many years, I've experienced the impact of changing my own diet and lifestyle. I've been through many of the struggles you've been through, but I'm also aware of the amazing results you'll experience if you stick with it.

I can be with you every step of the way to guarantee your success.

To book a call with me, so that we can explore how I can best help you, go to www.silvanahealthandnutrition.com/booking and follow the instructions to book your slot. Together, we can turn your 10 Day Sugar Detox Challenge into a long-term sugar-free life.

If you do choose to go it alone, I wish you all luck and success.

And lastly, if you enjoyed this book and found it helpful, please go to Amazon and leave a review. By doing this, we can reach out to more people and help them kick the sugar habit to lead a healthier life.

Lots of love xx

Silvana

About the Author

Silvana Siskov is the author of numerous books focusing on health, weight loss, and well-being. She is a dedicated health coach, counsellor, and nutritionist. Over the last two decades, she has focused her time and attention on helping her clients manage various problems, including weight loss, issues with confidence, stress, and other psychological and emotional issues. She has a deep-seated desire to help others and, through her work, has successfully done so.

When Silvana experienced her own health issues about 10 years ago, she found that focusing on self-care helped turn her health and life around. She started to feel full of energy and in a better place. By implementing some lifestyle changes, she became confident that she could help others do the same, and by doing so, they could improve their health and well-being.

The power of a healthy lifestyle comes from within. By giving sound advice on a healthy balanced diet and focusing on the power of sleep, exercise, and self-care, Silvana has helped countless people overcome chronic stress conditions and other health issues that negatively affected their lives.

With Silvana's strong background in psychology and her combined working and personal experience, she has empathy and understanding for her clients, which helps her connect with them on a deeper level so they can make positive and successful changes in their lives.

More recently, Silvana's books have made a big difference in her readers' lives, helping them with their weight loss issues, menopausal symptoms, emotional and binge eating, and generally having better health and improved well-being.

Helpful Resources

Books by Silvana Siskov:

- *"Get Your Sparkle Back: 10 Steps to Weight Loss and Overcoming Emotional Eating."* The book is available on Amazon. Go to http://viewbook.at/sparkle.
- *"Live Healthy on a Tight Schedule: 5 Easy Ways for Busy People to Develop Sustainable Habits Around Food, Exercise and Self-Care."* The book is available on Amazon. Go to http://viewbook.at/livehealthy.
- *"Get Fit and Healthy in Your Own Home in 20 Minutes or Less: An Essential Daily Exercise Plan and Simple Meal Ideas to Lose Weight and Get the Body You Want."* The book is available on Amazon. Go to http://viewbook.at/get-fit.
- *"Get Fit and Healthy on a Tight Schedule 2 Books in 1."* The book is available on Amazon. Go to http://viewbook.at/get-fit2books.
- *"Beat Your Menopause Weight Gain: Balance Hormones, Stop Middle-Age Spread, Boost Your Health And Vitality."* The book is available on Amazon. Go to http://viewbook.at/beat-menopause.
- *"Free Yourself From Hot Flushes and Night Sweats: The Essential Guide to a Happy And Healthy Menopause."* The book is available on Amazon. Go to http://viewbook.at/healthy-menopause.
- *"Manage Your Menopause 2 Books in 1: How to*

Balance Hormones and Prevent Middle-Age Spread." The book is available on Amazon. Go to http://viewbook.at/manage-menopause.

- *"Break the Binge Eating Cycle: Stop Self-Sabotage and Improve Your Relationship With Food."* The book is available on Amazon. Go to http://viewbook.at/breakthebinge.
- *"Relaxation and Stress Management Made Simple: 7 Proven Strategies to Calm Your Mind, Stop Negative Thinking and Improve Your Life."* The book is available on Amazon. Go to http://viewbook.at/stressfree.

Free Mini-Courses:

- *Discover 10 Secrets of Successful Weight Loss*
- *This is How to Start Eating Less Sugar*
- *Learn How to Boost Your Energy – 11 Easy Ways*
- *Your Guide to a Happy and Healthy Menopause*
- *This is How to Lose Weight in Your 40's and Beyond*

Free Mini-Courses Available at:

www.silvanahealthandnutrition.com/course/

To join the mailing list for updates on future books and to receive information about health, weight loss, and nutrition, please go to:

www.bit.ly/silvana-signup

References

1. *US children eat 3 times as much sugar as they should* (2016). Insider, https://www.businessinsider.com/afp-us-kids-eat-3x-times-too-much-added-sugar-health-group-2016-8?amp
2. Timsit, A. (2018). *American toddlers are eating more sugar than the maximum amount recommended for adults*, Quartz. https://qz.com/1302201/american-toddlers-are-eating-more-sugar-than-the-amount-recommended-for-adults/
3. *Diabetes Statistics* (n.d.). Diabetes UK. https://www.diabetes.org.uk/professionals/position-statements-reports/statistics
4. *National Diabetes Statistics Report* (2022). Centers for Disease Control and Prevention. https://www.cdc.gov/diabetes/data/statistics-report/index.html
5. Vass, A. (2002). Obesity causes 30.000 deaths a year, BMJ Publishing Group. https://www.ncbi.nlm.nih.gov/pmc/articles/PMC117 2013/
6. Hales, M.C., (M.D.), Carroll, D. M., (M.S.P.H.), Fryar, D., (M.S.P.H.), & Ogden, L., (Ph.D), (2022). *Prevalence of Obesity and Severe Obesity Among Adults: United States*, Centers for Disease Control and Prevention. https://www.cdc.gov/nchs/products/databriefs/db36

0.htm#:~:text=Examination%20Survey%20(NHANES)-
,What%20was%20the%20prevalence%20of%20obesit
y%20among%20adults%20in%202017,adults%20aged
%2060%20and%20over

7. Ahmed, S. H., Guillem, K., & Vandaele, Y. (2013). *Sugar addiction: pushing the drug-sugar analogy to the limit.* Current Opinion in Clinical Nutrition and Metabolic Care.https://journals.lww.com/co-clinicalnutrition/Abstract/2013/07000/Sugar_addicti on_pushing_the_drug_sugar_analogy_to.11.aspx

8. *How Sugar Is Made — The History,* (n.d.). Sugar Knowledge International Ltd. https://www.sucrose.com/lhist.html

9. Touger-Decker, R., & van Loveren, C. (2003). *Sugars and Dental Caries.* The American Journal of Clinical Nutrition. https://academic.oup.com/ajcn/article/78/4/881S/46 90063

10. Bovi, A. P. D., Michelle, L. D., Laino, G., & Vajro, P. (2017). *Obesity and Obesity Related Diseases, Sugar Consumption and Bad Oral Health: A Fatal Epidemic Mixtures.* The Pediatric and Odontologist Point of View. Translational Medicine @UniSa https://www.ncbi.nlm.nih.gov/pmc/articles/PMC553 6157/

11. Te Morenga, L.A., Howatson A.J., Jones, R.M., & Mann, J. (2014). *Dietary sugars and cardiometabolic risk: systematic review and meta-analyses of randomized controlled trials of the effects on blood pressure and lipids.* The American Journal of Clinical Nutrition. 100(1). 65–79. https://academic.oup.com/ajcn/article/100/1/65/45 76668

12. Avena, N. M., Rada, P., & Hoebel, B.G. (2007). *Evidence for sugar addiction: Behavioral and neurochemical*

effects of intermittent, excessive sugar intake. Neuroscience & Biobehavioral Reviews 32(1), 20-39. https://www.ncbi.nlm.nih.gov/entrez/eutils/elink.fcgi ?dbfrom=pubmed&retmode=ref&cmd=prlinks&id=17 617461

13. Harvard T.H. Chan School of Public Health (n.d.). *Low-Calorie Sweeteners.* https://www.hsph.harvard.edu/nutritionsource/healt hy-drinks/artificial-sweeteners/

14. Liu, A. G., Ford, N.A. & Kris-Etherton, P.M. (2017). *A healthy approach to dietary fats: understanding the science and taking action to reduce consumer confusion.* Nutrition Journal. https://www.ncbi.nlm.nih.gov/pmc/articles/PMC557776 6/

15. Australian Government, National Health and Medical Research Council (2014). *Macronutrient Balance,* https://www.nrv.gov.au/chronic-disease/macronutrient-balance

16. Rada, P., Avena, M.N., & Hoebel, G.B. (2005). *Daily bingeing on sugar repeatedly releases dopamine in the accumbens shell.* Neuroscience. 134 (3). 737-744. https://www.sciencedirect.com/science/article/abs/p ii/S0306452205004288?via%3Dihub

17. Harvard T.H. Chan School of Public Health (n.d.). *Mindful Eating.* https://www.hsph.harvard.edu/nutritionsource/mind ful-eating/

18. Colantuoni, C., Schwenker, J., McCarthy, J, Rada, P., Ladenheim, B., Cadet, J., Schwartz, G.J., Moran, T.H., & Hoebel, B.G. (2001). *Excessive sugar intake alters binding to dopamine and mu-opioid receptors in the brain.* NeuroReport. 12(16). 3549-3552. https://journals.lww.com/neuroreport/Abstract/200 1/11160/Excessive_sugar_intake_alters_binding_to_

dopamine.35.aspx

19. Yang. Q., (PhD), Zhang, Z., (MD), (PhD), & Gregg E. W. (2014). *Added Sugar Intake and Cardiovascular Disease Mortality Among US Adults*. Jama Network. https://jamanetwork.com/journals/jamainternalmedicine/fullarticle/1819573

20. DiSalvo, D., (2012). *What Eating Too Much Sugar Does to Your Brain*. Forbes. https://www.forbes.com/sites/daviddisalvo/2012/04/01/what-eating-too-much-sugar-does-to-your-brain/?sh=417425924a19

21. Colloca, S., (2017), *Uova al pomodoro piccante*. Delicious. https://www.delicious.com.au/recipes/uova-al-pomodoro-piccante-eggs-poached-spicy-tomato-sauce-del-sunday/wA87qn81?r=recipes/group/n6q1utfn

22. Yasin, K., (n.d.). *Overnight Oats*. Healthline. https://www.healthline.com/health/food-nutrition/sugar-free-breakfast-recipes#1.-overnight-oats

23. Gunst, K., (n.d.). *Smoked Salmon & Cream Cheese Omelet*. EatingWell. https://www.eatingwell.com/recipe/251375/smoked-salmon-cream-cheese-omelet/

24. *Really Green Smoothie*. (n.d.). EatingWell. https://www.eatingwell.com/recipe/270514/really-green-smoothie/

25. Yasin, K. (n.d.). *Broccoli Rabe & Egg Toast*. Healthline. https://www.healthline.com/health/food-nutrition/sugar-free-breakfast-recipes#4.-broccoli-rabe-egg-toast

26. *Hash Brown Potatoes Recipe*. (n.d.). Yummly. https://www.yummly.com/recipe/Hash-Brown-Potatoes-2663157

27. *Breakfast Salad with Egg & Salsa Verde Vinaigrette.* (2020). EatingWell. https://www.eatingwell.com/recipe/281188/breakfa st-salad-with-egg-salsa-verde-vinaigrette/

28. *Baby Kale Breakfast Salad with Smoked Trout & Avocado,* (2016). EatingWell. https://www.eatingwell.com/recipe/251411/baby-kale-breakfast-salad-with-smoked-trout-avocado/

29. Silva, J., (2019). *Salmon Quinoa Salad with Balsamic Vinaigrette.* A Sassy Spoon. https://asassyspoon.com/salmon-quinoa-salad/

30. *Glowing Spiced Lentil Soup.* (2016.). Oh She Glows. https://ohsheglows.com/2016/04/03/glowing-spiced-lentil-soup/

31. Lexis., (2017). *Mediterranean Tuna Salad with No Mayo!* Lexi's Clean Kitchen. https://lexiscleankitchen.com/mediterranean-tuna-salad/

32. *Golden Sun-Dried Tomato Red Lentil Pasta.* (2017). Half Baked Harvest. https://www.halfbakedharvest.com/golden-sun-dried-tomato-red-lentil-pasta/

33. PureWow Editors. (n.d.). *Chickpea and Vegetable Coconut Curry.* PureWow. https://www.purewow.com/recipes/chickpea-vegetable-coconut-curry

34. Bustard, D. (2019). *Turkey Taco Meal Prep Bowls.* Sweet Peas and Saffron. https://sweetpeasandsaffron.com/turkey-taco-lunch-bowls-meal-prep/

35. Melanie., (2016). *Mediterranean Chicken Wrap.* Nutritious Eats. http://www.nutritiouseats.com/mediterranean-chicken-wrap/

36. *Hearty Chickpea & Spinach Stew.* (2019). EatingWell.

https://www.eatingwell.com/recipe/270568/hearty-chickpea-spinach-stew/

37. Mathis, A., (2021). *Spinach & Artichoke Casserole with Chicken and Cauliflower Rice.* EatingWell. https://www.eatingwell.com/recipe/7916770/spinach-artichoke-casserole-with-chicken-and-cauliflower-rice/

38. Ramee, A., (2021). *Quinoa Chili with Sweet Potatoes.* EatingWell. https://www.eatingwell.com/recipe/7909910/quinoa-chili-with-sweet-potatoes/

39. *One Pot Pasta with Spinach & Mushrooms.* (2022). Simply Quinoa. https://www.simplyquinoa.com/one-pot-pasta-with-spinach/

40. *Beet Larb with Quinoa.* (n.d.). Punchfork. https://www.punchfork.com/recipe/Beet-Larb-with-Quinoa-EatingWell

41. Killeen, B. L., (2019) *Salt & Vinegar Sheet-Pan Chicken & Brussels Sprouts.* EatingWell. https://www.eatingwell.com/recipe/275788/salt-vinegar-sheet-pan-chicken-brussels-sprouts/

42. Loveless, S. E., (2019). *Slow-Cooker Mediterranean Diet Stew.* EatingWell. https://www.eatingwell.com/recipe/277511/slow-cooker-mediterranean-stew/

43. Cheng M., (2017). *Salmon & Avocado Poke Bowl.* EatingWell. https://www.eatingwell.com/recipe/257112/salmon-avocado-poke-bowl/

44. *One-Ingredient Watermelon Sorbet.* (n.d.). PureWow. https://www.purewow.com/recipes/One-Ingredient-Watermelon-Sorbet

45. Duggan, E., (2017). *Sugar-Free Chocolate & Sticky Date Pudding.* Delicious. https://www.delicious.com.au/recipes/sugar-free-

chocolate-sticky-date-pudding/aq57hjoz?r=recipes/collections/6rr2ruhe

46. Godwin S., (2016). *Banana Pancakes, BBC Good Food,* https://www.bbcgoodfood.com/recipes/banana-pancakes/amp

47. Jawad, Y., (2020). *Apple Chips.* (n.d.). Well Plated by Erin. https://www.wellplated.com/apple-chips/

48. Jawad, Y., (2020). Feel Good Foodie. *Date Shake.* FeelGoodFoodie. https://feelgoodfoodie.net/recipe/date-shake/

49. *Hot Chocolate with Superfoods.* (2020). The Healthy Maven. https://www.thehealthymaven.com/superfood-hot-chocolate/

50. Team, G. F. (n.d.). *Slow cooker rice pudding recipe | BBC Good Food.* BBC Good Food. https://www.bbcgoodfood.com/recipes/slow-cooker-rice-pudding

Made in the USA
Columbia, SC
09 November 2023

25829390R00104